AF667473

Hemophilia - Recent Advances

Edited by Pankaj Abrol

Published in London, United Kingdom

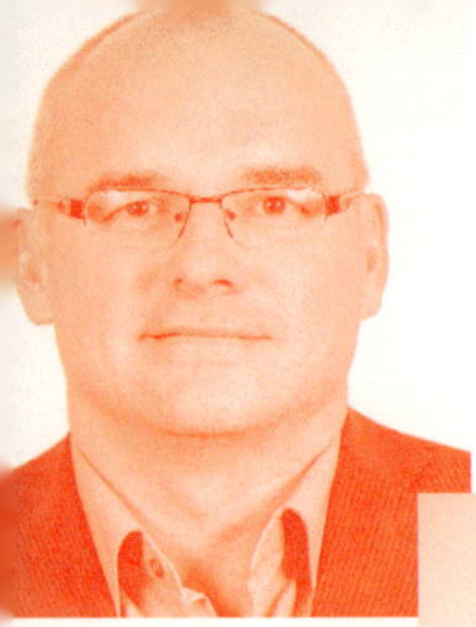

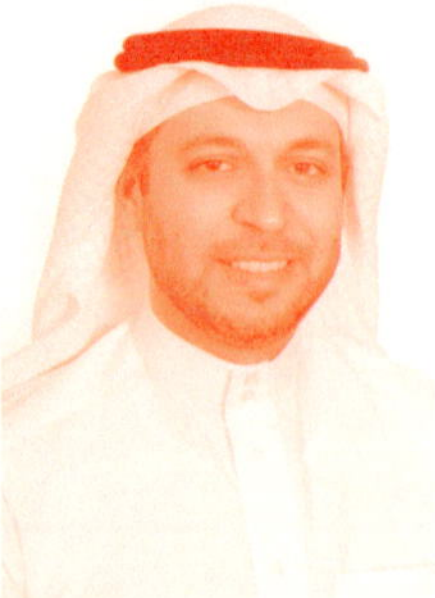

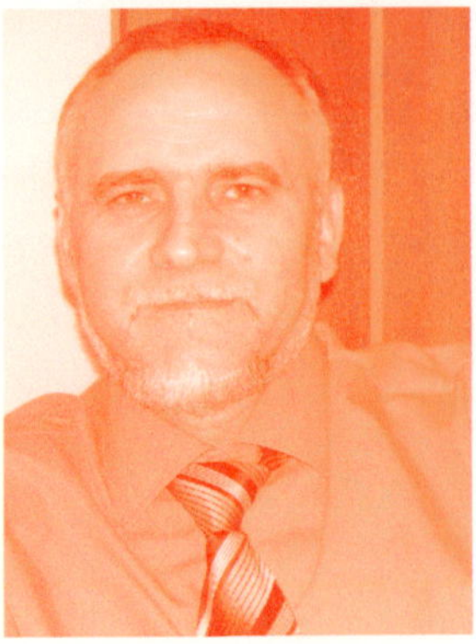

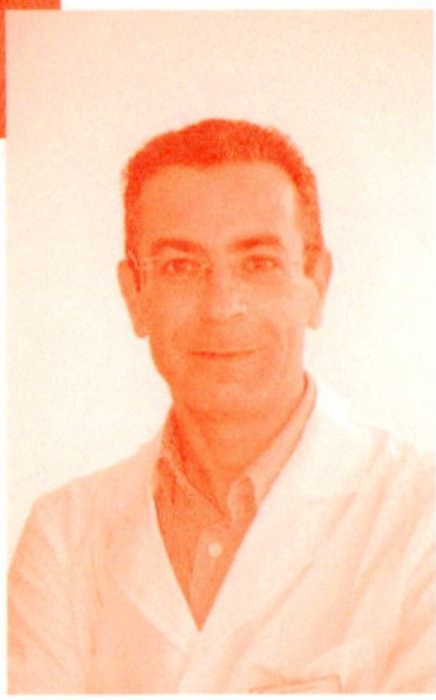

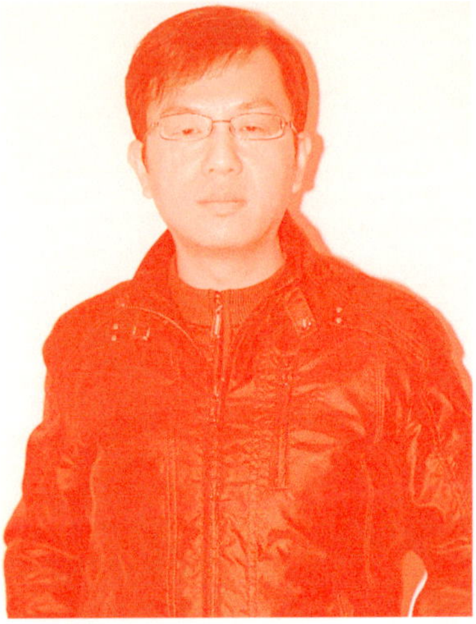

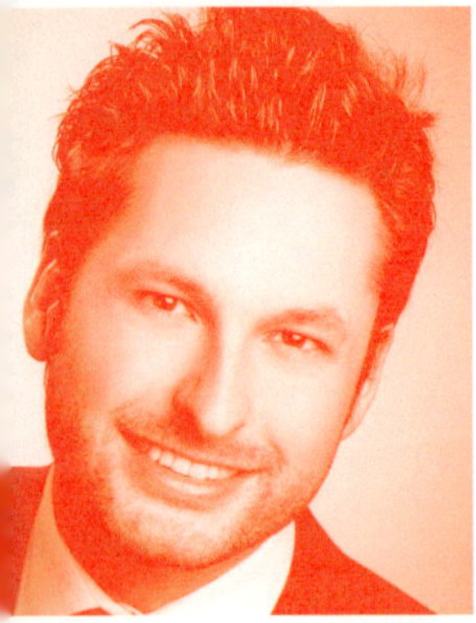

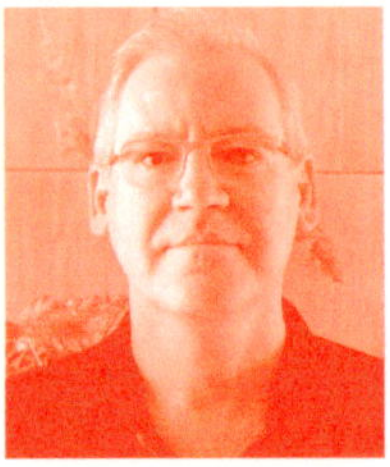

IntechOpen

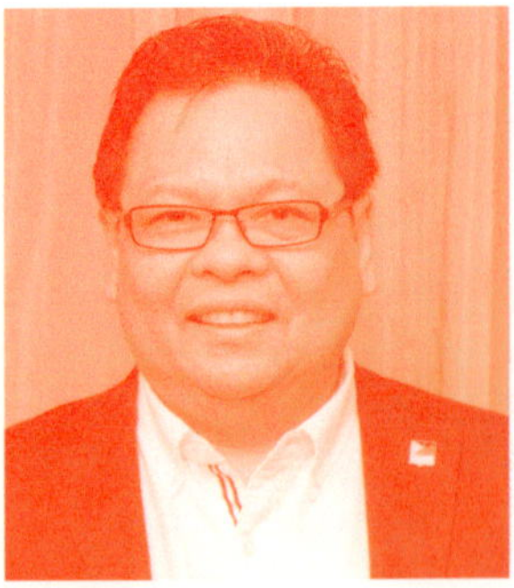

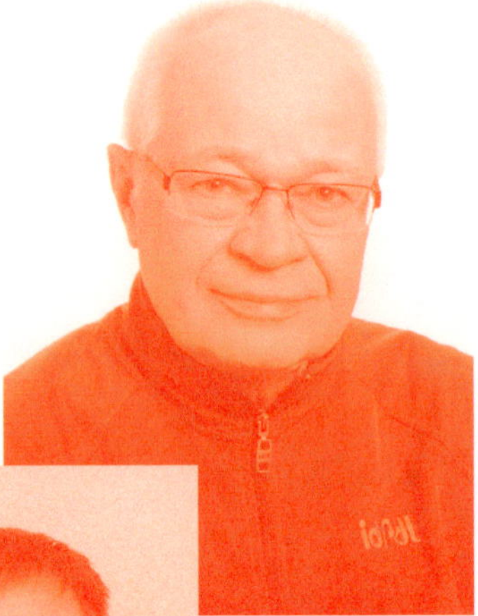

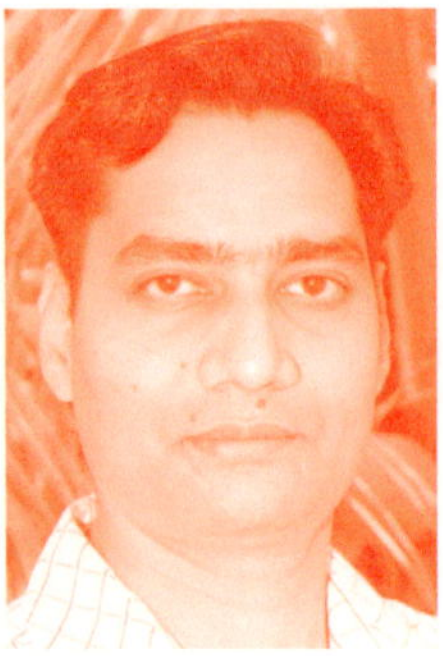

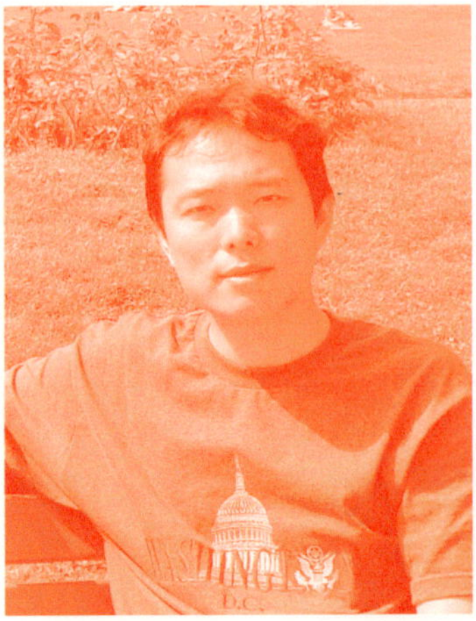

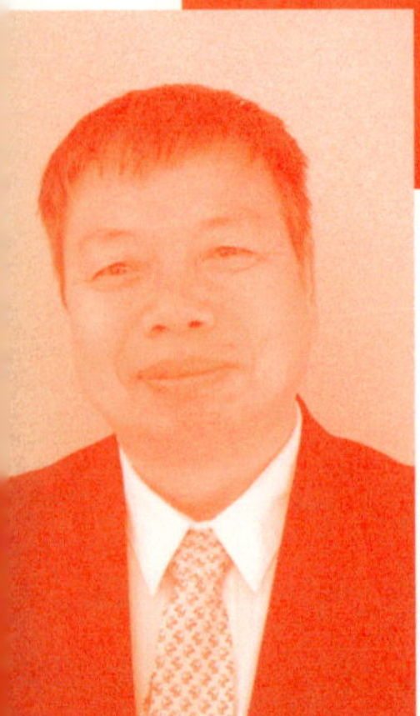

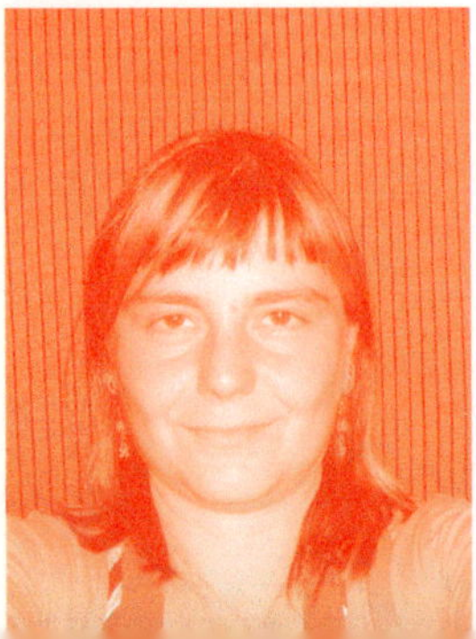

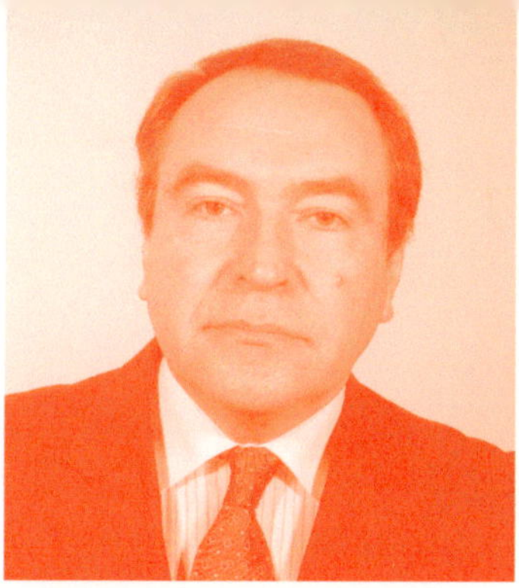
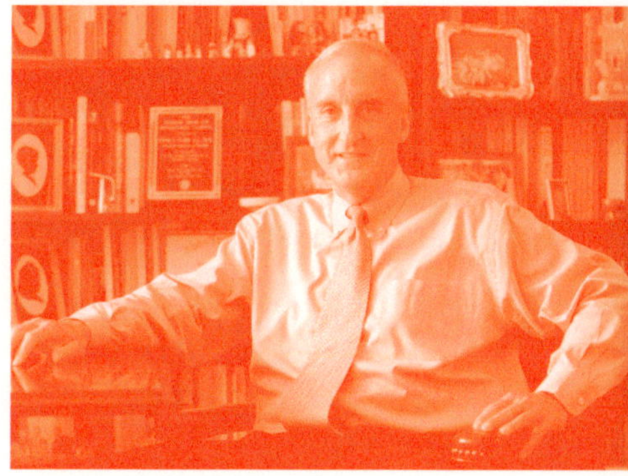
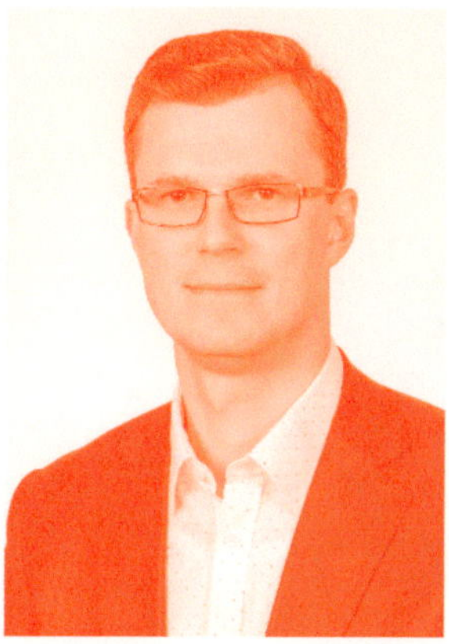
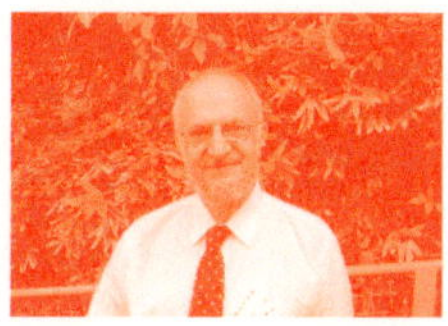
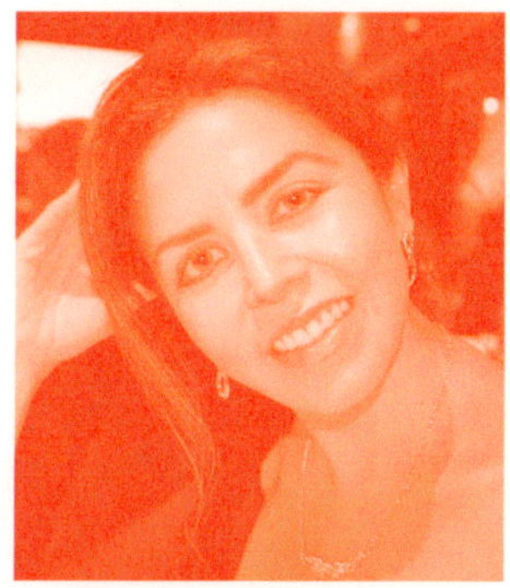

Supporting open minds since 2005

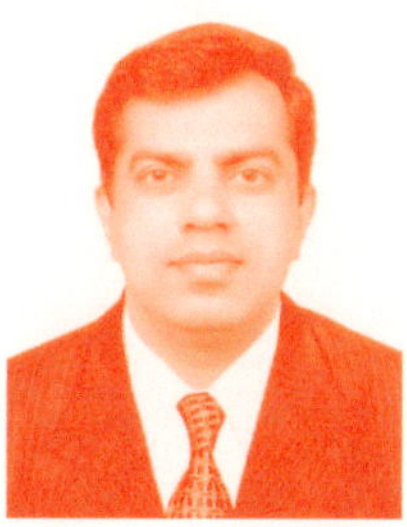
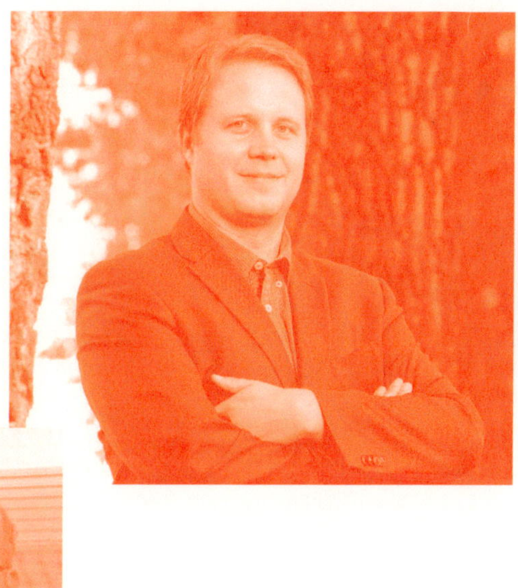
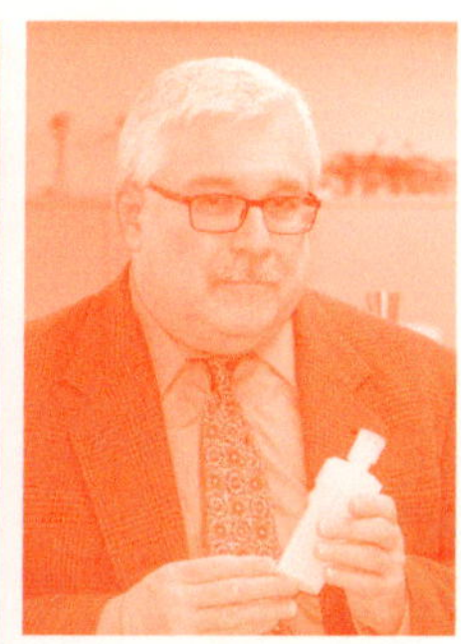
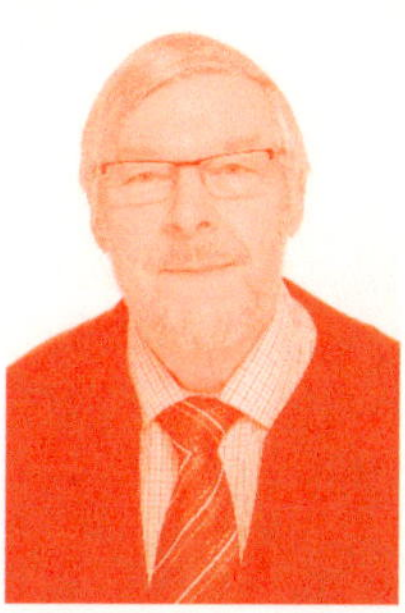
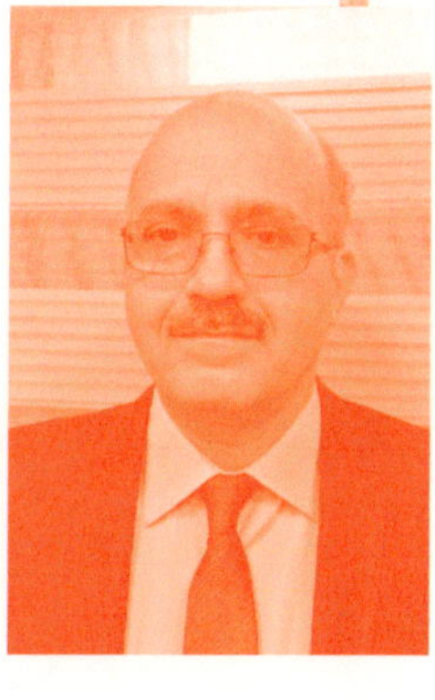
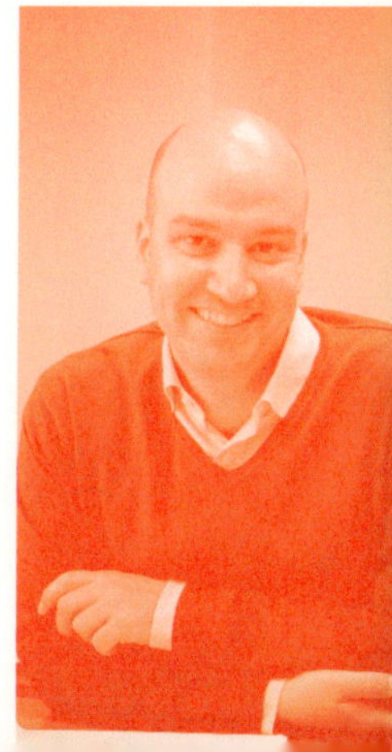
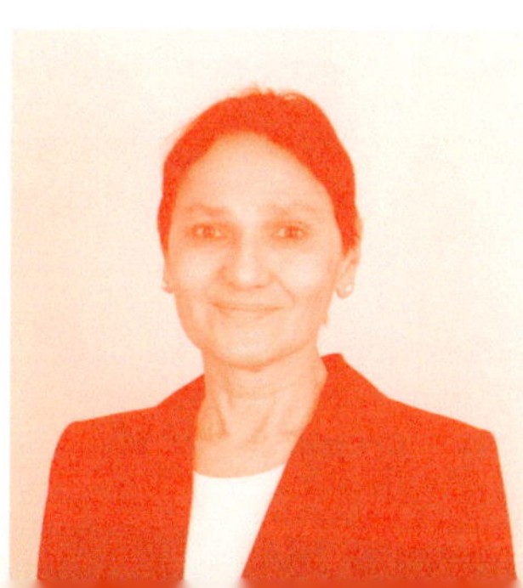

Hemophilia - Recent Advances
http://dx.doi.org/10.5772/intechopen.73877
Edited by Pankaj Abrol

Contributors
Muhammad Tariq Masood Khan, Abid Sohail Taj, Yasuhiro Maeda, Atsushi Okamoto, Kenta Yamamoto, Go Eguchi, Yoshitaka Kanai, Terufumi Yamaguchi, Ana Rebeca Jaloma-Cruz, Isaura-Araceli González-Ramos, Clara-Ibet Juárez-Vázquez, Diana Ornelas-Ricardo, Hilda Luna-Záizar, Pankaj Abrol

© The Editor(s) and the Author(s) 2019
The rights of the editor(s) and the author(s) have been asserted in accordance with the Copyright, Designs and Patents Act 1988. All rights to the book as a whole are reserved by INTECHOPEN LIMITED. The book as a whole (compilation) cannot be reproduced, distributed or used for commercial or non-commercial purposes without INTECHOPEN LIMITED's written permission. Enquiries concerning the use of the book should be directed to INTECHOPEN LIMITED rights and permissions department (permissions@intechopen.com).
Violations are liable to prosecution under the governing Copyright Law.

Individual chapters of this publication are distributed under the terms of the Creative Commons Attribution 3.0 Unported License which permits commercial use, distribution and reproduction of the individual chapters, provided the original author(s) and source publication are appropriately acknowledged. If so indicated, certain images may not be included under the Creative Commons license. In such cases users will need to obtain permission from the license holder to reproduce the material. More details and guidelines concerning content reuse and adaptation can be found at http://www.intechopen.com/copyright-policy.html.

Notice
Statements and opinions expressed in the chapters are these of the individual contributors and not necessarily those of the editors or publisher. No responsibility is accepted for the accuracy of information contained in the published chapters. The publisher assumes no responsibility for any damage or injury to persons or property arising out of the use of any materials, instructions, methods or ideas contained in the book.

First published in London, United Kingdom, 2019 by IntechOpen
IntechOpen is the global imprint of INTECHOPEN LIMITED, registered in England and Wales, registration number: 11086078, The Shard, 25th floor, 32 London Bridge Street
London, SE19SG - United Kingdom
Printed in Croatia

British Library Cataloguing-in-Publication Data
A catalogue record for this book is available from the British Library

Additional hard copies can be obtained from orders@intechopen.com

Hemophilia - Recent Advances
Edited by Pankaj Abrol
p. cm.
Print ISBN 978-1-78985-817-4
Online ISBN 978-1-78985-818-1

For EU product safety concerns:
IN TECH d.o.o., Prolaz Marije Krucifikse Kozulić 3, 51000 Rijeka, Croatia, info@intechopen.com or visit our website at intechopen.com.

We are IntechOpen, the world's leading publisher of Open Access books

Built by scientists, for scientists

4,100+
Open access books available

116,000+
International authors and editors

120M+
Downloads

151
Countries delivered to

Our authors are among the
Top 1%
most cited scientists

12.2%
Contributors from top 500 universities

CLARIVATE ANALYTICS BOOK CITATION INDEX INDEXED

WEB OF SCIENCE™

Selection of our books indexed in the Book Citation Index in Web of Science™ Core Collection (BKCI)

Interested in publishing with us?
Contact book.department@intechopen.com

Numbers displayed above are based on latest data collected.
For more information visit www.intechopen.com

Meet the editor

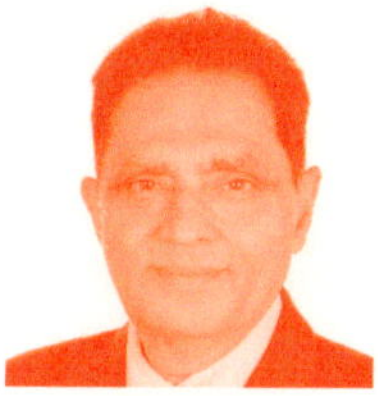

Dr. Pankaj Abrol is presently a professor and the head of the Department of Pediatrics, SGT Medical College Hospital & Research Institute, Gurgaon, India. He is a former senior professor and head of Pediatrics-II in the Postgraduate Institute of Medical Sciences, Rohtak, where he was Chief Pediatric Hematologist Oncologist, and in charge of Thalassemia & Hemophilia Day Care Centers. He is an active participant in the hemophilia training program in India and initiated free treatment of hemophilia with factors in the state of Haryana. He established a pediatric cancer unit after getting trained at Tata Memorial Hospital, Mumbai, India. He obtained the MBBS and MD (Pediatrics) degrees from the Institute of Medical Sciences, Banaras Hindu University, Varanasi. He is a resource person for pediatric oncology, thalassemia, and hemophilia at state as well as national level. He has many publications in the field and is a reviewer for various journals in pediatrics and pediatric hematology oncology. His exemplary services in the field of pediatrics and pediatric hematology oncology won him the Fellowship of Indian Academy of Pediatrics (FIAP). He has more than 35 years of experience teaching many graduates and postgraduates.

Contents

Preface

Hemophilia is a rare inherited disease due to a deficiency of coagulation factors VIII and IX. It was initially detected in the royal families of the UK, Russia, Spain, and Germany; hence, it is labeled a royal disease. Though known since biblical times, the term hemophilia was ascribed to Schonlein in the 1820s. Low levels of factor VIII were identified in 1947. Decreased levels of factor IX were shown in Hemophilia B in 1952. A lot of knowledge was acquired later and management progressed from plasma to FFP to cryoprecipitate to purified plasma-derived factors to recombinant factors—first, second, and third generation. There had been significant improvement in first aid measures for the management of multiple complications like arthropathy and the development of inhibitors. Improvement in treatment has seen various phases—from general therapy with plasma to specific therapy with recombinant factors. Now efforts are being made to prolong the half-life of factors VIII and IX to genetic therapy by targeting the affected gene.

It gives me immense pleasure to be associated with and edit a book on hemophilia, a disease for which research is making rapid advances. I have been associated with hemophilia for a long time and have organized hemophilia care in the state of Haryana in India and initiated steps for the free supply of factors VIII and IX for poor and needy patients.

This book covers various important aspects of hemophilia management. State-of-the-art chapters have been written by various authors. The chapter on genotype-phenotype correlation describes the changing concepts of multiple mutations in hemophilia and emphasizes the role of gene-environment interaction. In the chapter on the perioperative management of hemophilia A, authors have discussed intraoperative and postoperative factor replacement therapy in hemophilia A patients undergoing minor and major surgeries. Factor replacement in hemophilia is discussed in detail. Hemophilia A and B being X-linked disorders are by and large considered as strictly affecting the male population. The chapter on women's issues in inherited bleeding disorders highlights that a significant number of heavy menstrual bleeders can be hemophilia A and B carriers, in addition to more common causes of von Willebrand disease (VWD), platelet disorders, and some rare bleeding disorders. This can pose serious life threats, especially after surgery or postpartum.

This book on hemophilia highlights the latest literature and many important aspects of this disease. A few decades ago, little was known about hemophilia. At present, we are able to save many lives and also alleviate morbidity and prevent disability due to rapid advances in first aid measures, physical therapy, and prophylaxis. Prophylaxis will undoubtedly prove the turning point in hemophilia management.

I sincerely hope this book will provide a guide to students, scientists, and clinicians working in hemophilia, benefitting all of us.

Dr. Pankaj Abrol
Professor & Head,
Pediatric Hematologist Oncologist,
Department of Pediatrics,
SGT Medical College Hospital & Research Institute,
Gurgaon (Haryana),
India

Chapter 1

Introductory Chapter: Hemophilia

Pankaj Abrol

1. Introduction

Hemophilia disease is caused by deficiency of coagulation factors VIII and IX. Former is called hemophilia A (80–85%) whereas latter is labeled hemophilia B (10–15%). Hemophilia A and B are X-linked disorders, have common clinical presentation, with no racial predilection and are seen in all ethnic groups. The incidence is 1 in 5000 male births. A rare variety of hemophilia—hemophilia C or Rosenthal syndrome (factor XI deficiency) is seen in Jews of Ashkenazi descent. It is a milder form of hemophilia and because of autosomal transmission affects both the sexes. As per annual global surveys by WFH number of PWH (people with hemophilia) is approximately 400,000 [1].

1.1 Pathophysiology

Factors VIII and IX along with phospholipid and calcium activate factor activating complex. This factor X activating complex or factor VII in presence of tissue factor activate factor IX initiating coagulation cascade. In laboratory prothrombin time (PT) measures activation of factor X by factor VII and is therefore normal in hemophilia.

After any injury, initial hemostatic response of the human body is to form a platelet plug and formation of fibrin clot to stop bleeding. In hemophilia clot formation is delayed. The clot is soft and not robust. Bleeding in open space leads to hemorrhage and significant blood loss. Bleeding in closed joint leads to tamponade effect. When the soft clot is lysed, rebleeding can occur following minimal trauma.

1.2 Classification

Hemophilia is classified as per baseline level of factors VIII or IX in blood. One unit is defined as amount present in 1 mL of normal plasma. Severe hemophilia means that coagulation factor is <1% of normal activity, i.e., <1 U/dL of plasma. Moderate hemophilia is between 1 and 5% of normal coagulant activity, i.e., 1–5 U/dL of plasma. And mild hemophilia when coagulant activity is higher than 5% of the activity, i.e., >5–40 U/dL of plasma.

1.3 Clinical presentation

Factor VIII and IX cannot cross placenta. So a neonate can bleed at birth or even a fetus can have bleeding in utero. Thirty percent of hemophilia patients may bleed after circumcision. Up to 3% may have ICH or intracranial hemorrhage [2], and half the number getting ECH (extracranial hemorrhage). Some may get ICH as well as ECH. All efforts should be made to prevent head trauma during delivery and discourage forceps or vacuum extraction. Mostly hemophilia is suspected at birth because of family history but in one-third, it may be due to spontaneous mutation and therefore giving no clue from family history.

When a toddler tries to cruise, he starts getting symptoms like easy bruising following minor traumas, hematomas and bleeding in to joints. In early years when child tries to stand and walk, ankle joint followed by knee joint become the target joint for bleeding and hemarthrosis becomes main symptom He may also bleed from mouth because of torn frenulum. By 1 year of age 90% hemophiliacs present with excessive bleeding [3]. In older children and adolescents hemarthrosis in knee and elbow joints becomes more common and these joints become target joints. Hinged joints like ankle knee and elbow are more often involved. In 70–80% of cases, hemarthrosis is the main presentation. Bleeding into muscles occurs in 10–20%. Less than 5% bleed in CNS. At the time of bleeding in joints, there is feeling of tingling or warmth. This is followed by increasing pain and loss of motion. In a younger child pain and swelling of the joints present earlier but as the child grows older and bleeding occurs in the joints, pain and swelling of joint decreases. The patient comes to know of bleeding earlier. They are able to tell their parents that they are bleeding in to joints and the treatment should be started. When a child continues to have repeated hemarthrosis, chronic effusion and hyperemia appears in joints. If not managed properly with coagulation factors, chronic arthropathy occurs. As the age advances more PWH (people with hemophilia) get crippled because of repeated hemarthrosis in resource restrained countries [4]. Hemophilia patients may also present with hematuria or GIT bleeding.

MUSCLES: hemophilia patients bleed deep inside muscles and these hematomas are difficult to palpate. The patient gets vague feeling of pain on movement and there is increase in circumference of the affected limb. If not managed properly it can lead to fibrosis and contractures with muscular atrophy and pseudotumor formation. Bleeding in to iliopsoas muscle is particularly notorious. Such a patient has vague pain and discomfort in lower abdomen and upper part of thigh, with internally rotated thigh. These patients may have massive internal hemorrhage in the muscles requiring urgent specific aggressive management with factors for a fortnight followed prophylaxis for several months [2].

1.4 Life-threatening hemorrhages in hemophilia

1. Bleeding in CNS.

2. Bleeding in and around airway.

3. All exsanguinating hemorrhages including bleeding in iliopsoas muscles.

Bleeding in CNS and around airway can cause pressure symptoms in vital areas and airway compression. Exsanguinating hemorrhages can also cause shock and death. Such episodes require urgent therapy on slightest suspicion.

1.5 Hemophilia in female carriers

Because of lyonization of X chromosome, some female hemophilia carriers have sufficient reduction in level of factor VIII or IX and have mild bleeding disorder. Carriers with factor level of 40–60% may have bleeding tendency [5]. Levels of factor VIII or IX should be determined in all these carriers to determine the need for treatment when they go for surgery or have bleeding episode. There is also 50% probability of birth of female hemophilia patient when a male hemophilia patient marries a female hemophilia carrier.

1.6 Laboratory evaluation

It is easy to diagnose severe hemophilia. Prothrombin time (PT) is normal and partial thromboplastin time (PTT) is 2–3 times prolonged. Mild hemophilia is difficult to diagnosis as PTT may be normal or slightly prolonged. In a newborn, PTT may be slightly prolonged due to deficiency of vitamin K dependent factor IX and raised level of factor VIII due to stress of delivery. So diagnosis of hemophilia may require repeated tests of coagulation times.

Diagnosis of factor IX deficiency is more difficult as available commercial PTT reagents are more sensitive to factor VIII deficiency. PTT may be normal even with factor IX level as low as 15–20 U/dL. So it is advisable to perform factor IX assay even when PTT is normal in suspected hemophilia B. Specific functional assays of factors VIII and IX are done by mixing studies to confirm the diagnosis of hemophilia A and B. When mixed 1:1 with normal plasma PTT becomes normal in hemophilia. If PTT is not corrected, one should suspect presence of inhibitors to factor VIII or IX. Other causes are presence of lupus inhibitor or heparin. If inhibitors are present, quantitative Bethesda assay should be performed to measure antibody titer.

Immunoassays of factors VIII and IX can also be done to identify dysfunctional proteins called cross-reacting material (CRM). Immunoassays are usually not required for management of hemophilia patients. Clot waveform analysis and thrombin generation assay are also recommended for accurate estimation of factor VIII and IX activity during management of hemophilia patients especially when the factor levels are very low [6].

1.7 Genetic testing

Both hemophilia A and B are X-linked traits, and the encoding genes F8 and F9 map to the distal portion of long arm of chromosomes [7]. Commonest genetic alteration is inversion and mostly originating in male germ cells. Family history is present in approximately two third of patients and mutations constitute one third of cases. Genetic resting is available and performed on proband first. African Americans have different haplotype and therefore have higher level of inhibitor formation. Prenatal testing can be done by amniocentesis or chorionic villous biopsy. Factor IX gene is smaller. Missense point mutation is seen in more than 60% of patients. In case genetic testing is not helping, coagulation based assay can also be used to detect carrier state and it is 90% accurate [8].

1.8 Treatment

Hallmark of treatment is prompt and appropriate management of bleeding episode; and prophylactic therapy to prevent future hemorrhages decreasing the incidence of chronic complications.

Supportive care: In general hemophilia patients should be advised to avoid trauma, but it is very difficult to advise a child in growing age of activity to completely do so. They can be advised to avoid risk prone behavior, use seat belts and bike helmets while driving. Ask them to avoid contact sports like, boxing and wrestling. They can do swimming and play table tennis, badminton, etc. In mild and moderate hemophilia these measures may help but in severe hemophilia there can be bleeding without trauma. Psychosocial counseling may help the child to achieve a balance. Hemophiliacs should be advised to avoid nonsteroidal anti-inflammatory drugs like aspirin, as these drugs interfere with platelet functions and aggregation, making him prone to bleeding. These patients should be immunized against hepatitis B and those on plasma-derived products should be screened periodically for HIV, hepatitis B and C.

Half-life of factor VIII is 8–12 h and that of factor IX is 18–24 h. In event of mild to moderate hemorrhage, level of factor VIII or IX has to be raised to hemostatic level of 35–50% range. In life threatening or severe hemorrhage, hemostatic level of factor should be raised to 100% [3].

Dose of recombinant factor VIII (rFVIII) in IU:

$$\text{Body weight (kg)} \times 0.5 \times \text{\%age of desired rise in rFVIII.} \tag{1}$$

Dose of recombinant factor IX (rFIX) in IU:

$$\text{Body weight (kg)} \times 1.4 \times \text{\%age of desired rise in rFIX.} \tag{2}$$

Endogenous factor VIII can be released by desmopressin acetate (DDAVP, 1-deamino-8-*d*-arginine vasopressin) in mild hemophilia. Intranasal preparation of concentrated preparation of desmopressin acetate 150 μg/puff is given as one puff to the patient weighing <50 kg and two puffs (300 μg) to patient >50 kg. Desmopressin is not effective in hemophilia B.

1.9 Recombinant factors

Development of recombinant factors is a major advance in treatment of hemophilia patients. Three generations—first, second and third generations are currently available [9]. First generation factor concentrates are stabilized with human albumin, second generation is stabilized with sucrose, and third generation is stabilized with/without additional human or animal plasma proteins. Efforts are still being made to get better recombinant factors with longer half-life and less immunogenicity, so that the frequency of prophylactic infusion may be further decreased [10]. With use of plasma derived factors, inhibitor formation is less, and after 150 EDs (exposure days) inhibitor formation is negligible [11]. In some centers, initial prophylaxis is given with plasma derived factors VIII and IX, and with recombinant factors after 150 EDs. Recombinant factor VIII is available in all three generations, but for factor IX, only third generation recombinant factor is available.

1.10 Adjunctive management

1. More important in resource limited conditions, when there is less availability of factor VIII and IX.

2. First aid measures are important in management of acute bleeding episode presenting as musculoskeletal hemorrhage like hemarthrosis. Protection (splint), rest, ice, compression and elevation (**PRICE**) are very useful in acute hemarthrosis [12].

3. Pain killers: NSAID drugs like aspirin should be avoided. Paracetamol is safest analgesic. Some COX-2 inhibitors can be judiciously used in arthropathy.

4. Physiotherapy/rehabilitation after pain decreases.

5. Antifibrinolytic drugs like tranexamic acid and epsilon aminocaproic acid can be used in mucosal bleeds and dental extraction.

1.11 Long-term complications

These are chronic arthropathy, development of inhibitors to factors VIII or IX and the risk of transfusion-transmitted infections.

a. Chronic arthropathy: hemarthrosis in target joints is commonest presentation in hemophilia. After every such episode, proteolytic enzymes are released by white blood cells in the joint space. Heme released from blood induces macrophage proliferation leading to synovitis. Thickened synovium develops frond like projections which on getting pinched induces further hemorrhage. Cartilaginous surface of the affected joint gets eroded and exposes bone surface leading to articular fusion and ankylosis. Because of repeated hemarthrosis, synovium gets more and more thickened leading to narrowing of joint space, little space to accommodate more blood and causing intense pain. Such patients need to be put on short-term or long-term prophylaxis to prevent progression of arthropathy.

b. Development of inhibitors: repeated infusion of factors VIII or IX may induce immune response leading to formation of inhibitor antibodies to the deficient factor. Such patients fail to respond to appropriate factor replacement after bleeding episode. Incidence of inhibitor development may be as high as 25–30% in hemophilia A and somewhat lower in hemophilia B. Risk of development of inhibitors is minimal after 150 exposure days to coagulation factors. MASAC (USA) advises inhibitor assay only up to 150 exposure days [11]. With recombinant factor VIII incidence of inhibitor development is 87% higher and 69% higher incidence of high titer inhibitor compared to plasma derived factors. Some inhibitors to factor IX may also cause anaphylaxis. Incidence of development of inhibitors is higher with recombinant factors than plasma derived factors. Such patients may lose inhibitors and respond after continued administration of factors. Some others may require desensitization by infusing higher dose of factor VIII or IX, saturating antibodies and inducing immune tolerance induction. Alternatives are rituximab, steroids and cyclophosphamide. In patients who do not respond to these agents, recombinant factor VIIa or prothrombin complex concentrate may be used to bypass factor VIII.

c. Risk of transfusion transmitted infections: in past, there had been many incidences of transmission of hepatitis B and C and even HIV when plasma derived factors VIII and IX were used. Now with advent of recombinant factors VIII and IX, such a risk is minimal but one must immunize these patients for hepatitis B and monitor immunization status of the patient.

Hemophilia A patients with inhibitors: these patients can be divided in to two types.

a. Low responding factor VIII inhibitors: inhibitor titer is <5 Bethesda units. These can be treated with factor VIII at higher doses. Continuous administration of factor VIII is more effective. For common muscle and joint hemorrhages, double dose of factor VIII is usually effective.

b. High responding factor VIII inhibitors: inhibitor titer is more than five Bethesda units. Requires management in a tertiary hemophilia care centers by hemophilia experts. Treatment is more aggressive. Alternatives are porcine factor VIII concentrates, recombinant factor VIIa, prothrombin complex concentrate or activated prothrombin complex concentrate (commercially available FEIBA or factor VIII inhibitor bypassing activity).

Hemophilia B patients with inhibitors: incidence of inhibitor formation is much lower but can cause anaphylaxis. Activated prothrombin complex concentrate and recombinant factor VII are very effective. In patients who have developed anaphylaxis, use of activated prothrombin complex concentrate is contraindicated as this contains some factor IX, use of factor VIIa is the answer [2]. Immune tolerance is not effective as some of the patients develop nephrotic syndrome if higher dose of factor IX is given.

1.12 Hemophilia prophylaxis

Hemophilia prophylaxis is regular administration of factors VIII or IX to the patient to prevent bleeding. It was observed that mid and moderate hemophilia patients, who have coagulation factor level >1% rarely had spontaneous hemorrhage. And if we can maintain factors VIII or IX level >1%, patient will not have spontaneous hemorrhage, thereby decreasing moribund and debilitating complications with much better preservation of joint functions. Prophylaxis requires insertion of central catheter to ensure venous access, is expensive, requires more of costly factors but reduces complications and preserves joints. Hemophilia prophylaxis can be primary, secondary or tertiary [9].

a. Primary regular prophylaxis: prophylaxis treatment started regularly before second clinically relevant large joint bleed and before 3 years of age. There is no documented osteochondral joint disease on clinical and radiological examination.

b. Secondary regular prophylaxis: prophylaxis treatment after two or more joint bleeds in to large joints and before the onset of joint disease, confirmed by clinical and radiological examination.

c. Tertiary regular prophylaxis: prophylaxis treatment after onset of joint disease documented after clinical and/or plain radiograph of affected joint.

Prophylaxis can also be classified as intermittent or continuous:

a. Intermittent (Periodic): prophylactic factors given for periods not exceeding 45 weeks in a year.

b. Continuous: with an intent to treat for 52 weeks/year and for at least 45 weeks (85%) of the year under consideration.

In a patient with repeated hemarthrosis or bleeding, short-term prophylaxis for 4–8 weeks is recommended to interrupt the bleeding cycle. Whether adults require long-term prophylaxis is not yet clear. More studies are required to confirm this. Some young adults can do well off prophylaxis. Prophylaxis does not reverse the damage already done to the affected joint, but it slows the progression of arthropathy and improves quality of life. It is also cost-effective as it helps to avoid the subsequent costly management of damaged joints.

Dose schedule for prophylaxis [12]:

a. Malmo protocol: 25–40 IU/kg per dose thrice a week for hemophilia A and twice a week for hemophilia B.

b. Utrecht protocol: 15–30 IU/kg per dose thrice a week for hemophilia A and twice a week for hemophilia B.

Many countries follow different protocols. Protocol should be individualized. It is best given in the morning to cover activity of whole day.

1.13 Home therapy of hemophilia

With home therapy treatment is started earlier, so onset of complications is delayed. A certificate program shall be helpful. Family and patient need to be educated about general information and perspective of hemophilia. They need to know about first aid measures; dosage calculation, storage and administration of coagulation factors. Knowledge about aseptic technique, central catheters, proper storage and disposal of needles, record keeping and management of blood spills is mandatory. Comprehensive care team should monitor all this by making frequent follow up visits. Family members should be motivated to take care of young children. Older children and young adults can learn self-infusion and care.

1.14 Comprehensive hemophilia treatment centers (CHTC)

Hemophilia treatment centers must provide comprehensive medical care to hemophilia patients. Multiple disciplines should be involved providing state of art medical care. The center should have hematologist, pediatrician, nurses, dentist, psychologist, social worker, physical therapist and orthopedist. Even patients and their families should be part of the team. Every year the patient should be assessed for individual and potential problems, so that if required his treatment can be modified.

Author details

Pankaj Abrol
Department of Pediatrics, Pediatric Hematologist Oncologist, SGT Medical College Hospital and Research Institute, Gurgaon, Haryana, India

*Address all correspondence to: abrolpankaj1@gmail.com

IntechOpen

© 2019 The Author(s). Licensee IntechOpen. This chapter is distributed under the terms of the Creative Commons Attribution License (http://creativecommons.org/licenses/by/3.0), which permits unrestricted use, distribution, and reproduction in any medium, provided the original work is properly cited.

References

[1] Stonebraker JS, Bolton-Maggs PH, Sourice JM, Walker I, Brooker M. A study of variations in reported hemophilia A prevalence around the world. Hemophilia. 2010;**16**(1):20-32

[2] Paula JD, Montgomery RR, Gill JC, Flood V. Hemophilia and von Willebrand disease. In: Nathan and Oski's Hematology and Oncology of Infancy and Childhood. 8th ed. Philadelphia: Elsevier Saunders; 2015. pp. 1028-1054

[3] Scott JP, Flood VH. Hereditary clotting factor deficiencies (bleeding disorders). In: Nelson Textbook of Pediatrics. 20th ed. Philadelphia: Elsevier; 2015. pp. 2384-2389

[4] Kar A, Mirkazemi R, Singh P, Potnis-Lele M, Lohade S, Lalwani A, et al. Disability in Indian patients with haemophilia. Hemophilia. 2007;**13**(4):398-404

[5] Plug I, Eveline P, Mauser-Bunschoten EP, Annette HJ, Brocker-Vriends AH, Hans KP, et al. Bleeding in carriers of hemophilia. Blood. 2006;**108**(1):52-56

[6] Matsumoto T, Shima M, Takeyama M, Yoshida K, Tanaka I, Sakurai Y, et al. The measurement of low level of factor VIII or factor IX in hemophilia A and hemophilia B plasma by clot waveform analysis and thrombin generation assay. Journal of Thrombosis and Haemostasis. 2006;**4**:377-384

[7] Goodeve AC, Perry DJ, Cumming T, et al. Genetics of haemostasis. Haemophilia. 2012;**18**(Suppl 4):73-80

[8] Graw J, Brackmann H, Oldenberg J, et al. Hemophilia A: From mutations analysis to new therapies. Nature Reviews. Genetics. 2005;**6**:488-501

[9] Morfini M, Coppola A, Franchini M, Minno GD. Clinical use of factor VIII and factor IX concentrates. Blood Transfusion. 2013;**11**(Suppl 4):s55-s63

[10] Lieuw K. Many factor VIII products available in the treatment of hemophilia A: An embarrassment of riches? Journal of Blood Medicine. 2017;**8**:67-73

[11] Hermans C, Astermark J, de Moerloose P. Exposure to factor VIII and prediction of inhibitor development: Exposure days vs. danger days, or both? Journal of Thrombosis and Haemostasis. 2012;**10**:2194-2196

[12] Srivastava A, Brewer AK, Mauser-Bunschoten EP, et al. Blackwell Publishing Ltd; 2012. [Epub Jul 6, 2012]

Chapter 2

Genotype-Phenotype Heterogeneity in Haemophilia

Muhammad Tariq Masood Khan and Abid Sohail Taj

Abstract

Haemophilia was previously regarded as a classical example of Mendelian inheritance, with mutation in only a single gene (F8 or F9) causing the disease phenotype. The disease manifests complete penetrance. Studies, however, revealed the striking genetic and phenotypic heterogeneities of the disease. With further sophistication of clinical and molecular techniques, the disease was also found to have allele heterogeneity, phenotypic plasticity and variation in expressivity. The variations are more pronounced in F9 variants with five distinct phenotypes. All these phenomena advocate a rather complex genotype-phenotype relationship for the disease. A keen insight into the matter may unveil new avenues of therapeutics.

Keywords: genotype-phenotype correlation, genotype-phenotype heterogeneity, haemophilia

1. Phenotypic variation

1.1 Background

A phenotype is defined as an observable characteristic which is expressed by an underlying genotype interacting with the environment [1]. Phenotype, in clinical scenario, hence represents the observable interface of the disease in terms of clinical features (laboratory findings, signs and symptoms) [2]. In contrast to genotype which is a stable entity, phenotype is dynamic and influenced by both the genotype and environment [3, 4]. Hence, in strict terms, the exact disease phenotype may be difficult to ascertain in many cases. This uncertainty usually underlies contemporary processes, directly or indirectly affecting the disease, with their own genetic and/or environmental influences [2]. Precise definition for a specific phenotype, therefore, needs development of a standardised comprehensive checklist of signs, symptoms and laboratory findings [3]. This is considerably convenient in case of monogenic disorders. Phenotypes for multigenic disorders or genetic diseases significantly influenced by environmental interactions are difficult to delineate [5].

1.2 Phenotypic variation in haemophilia

Haemophilia is known to mankind since ancient times with references from Babylonian history [6]. The first vague description of cases appeared in the tenth century [7]. The first modern description of the disease was made in the eighteenth century, and the term haemophilia was first used in 1828 by Johann Lukas Schönlein and his student Friedrich Hopff [6].

The two diseases, haemophilia A (HA) and haemophilia B (HB), were initially regarded as the same and attributed to fragility of vessels [8]. The idea later shifted to abnormalities in platelets in the 1930s. It was in 1937, when Patek and Taylor found the 'anti-haemophilic globulin', extracted from plasma, to be the factor responsible. The two diseases were, however, first discriminated in 1944 by Pavlosky of Buenos Aires [8].

In haemophilia, the phenotype is expressed at three distinct levels: the coagulation activity, the factor antigen level and the clinical outcome in terms of bleeding and its complications. Plasma procoagulant level, determined by coagulation activity, is the most important clinical entity determining severity of the disease. Employing this parameter, the Scientific and Standardisation Committee classified haemophilia A and haemophilia B into three major classes, that is, mild, moderate and severe [9]. Each phenotype has a distinct clinical impact (**Table 1**). Patients with severe phenotype (plasma factor level < 0.01 IU/ml; <1% of normal) commonly present with frequent (two to five bleeding episodes per month) spontaneous bleeding into the joints or deep muscles. Patients with moderate severity of the disease (plasma factor level 0.01–0.05 IU/ml; 1–5% of normal) would bleed following mild trauma; spontaneous bleeding is seen uncommonly. Diagnosis is usually established in the first 5–6 years of life. Bleeding frequency ranges from once a month to once a year. In mild severity of the disease (plasma factor level >0.05 to <0.40 IU/ml; >5 to <40% of normal), bleeding occurs as a result of major trauma, e.g., surgery or accident. Bleeding is infrequent in these patients [10, 11].

This is, however, noteworthy that patients with a specific severity of the disease do not always behave as anticipated. Studies have reported a significant number of severe haemophilia cases with a milder phenotype [1, 12, 13]. In such cases, bleeding phenotype resembles that of moderate severity. These cases are hence treated like moderate haemophilia; prophylactic treatment is often not needed.

Severity	FVIII:C/FIX:C level (%)	Age at diagnosis	Bleeding and haemarthroses
Severe	≤1	≤2 years	Spontaneous haemorrhages and haemarthroses since early childhood
Moderate	2–5	<6 years	Haemorrhage are usually secondary to minor trauma or surgery; spontaneous haemarthrosis is unusual
Mild	6–40	Subject to haemostatic challenge	Haemorrhage secondary to surgery or major trauma; spontaneous bleedings are rare

FVIII:C, factor VIII coagulation activity; FIX:C, factor IX coagulation activity.

Table 1.
Haemophilia severity classification on the basis of FVIII:C/FIX:C levels.

2. Genetic heterogeneity in haemophilia

Haemophilia was previously regarded as a classical example of Mendelian inheritance, with mutation in only one gene (F8 or F9) causing the disease phenotype. The concept, however, has significantly evolved in the last couple of decades, and the two diseases are now recognised to have a heterogeneous spectrum of mutations. More than 2800 mutations are reported in F8, whereas more than 1200

Mutation type	F8	F9
Missense/nonsense	1674	748
Splicing	193	101
Regulatory	10	28
Small deletions	489	161
Small insertions	160	52
Small indels	38	17
Gross deletions	260	75
Gross insertions/duplications	40	7
Complex rearrangements	20	13
Repeat variations	0	0
Total	**2884**	**1202**

F8, factor VIII gene; F9, factor IX gene.

Table 2.
Frequency of different types of mutations reported in F8 and F9.

mutations are reported in F9 [14]. These mutations, summarised in **Table 2**, include all the major types of mutations. Point mutations are the most frequent, followed by small indel mutations. Repeat variants are not yet reported to associate with the disease. In majority of the cases, specific mutations result in the same disease severity, a phenomenon referred to as genotype-phenotype correlation [13, 15].

2.1 Disease penetrance and expressivity

Penetrance refers to the appearance of disease in affected individuals, whereas expressivity is the degree of severity of disease in patients [16]. Haemophilia is an X-linked recessive genetic disorder with complete penetrance in most of the cases, that is, male individuals with pathogenic variants in F8 or F9 are mostly fated to have haemophilia. This stands true particularly in case of F8. Patients from the same family have approximately the same severity status. However, the severity, as described earlier, is not the same in all patients. Cases with the same mutations exhibiting different levels of coagulation factor activity advocate variable expressivity for the specific genotype. This variation is believed to be the outcome factors including genetic alterations or polymorphisms in other genes (especially those related to haemostasis, inflammation and immune response) and environmental factors [17]. It has been established that the same genotype subjected to different environments expresses diverse phenotypes [18]. This interaction between genotype and environment is called gene–environment interaction [19, 20].

Large structural changes in the protein, by default, tend to generate a severe phenotype. Nonsense mutations, particularly those occurring in the early gene segments, have a similar tendency. Almost all the nonsense mutations reported within the initial part of the gene are associated with severe disease phenotype. Frameshift mutations in F8/F9 gene are again usually associated with an adverse phenotype [21].

Approximately 30% of the female individuals with heterozygous mutation have a coagulation factor activity less than 40% [22]. Increased bleeding tendency among the carriers, in comparison to normal females, is well documented [23, 24].

In case of F9 sequence variants, besides classical HB, four other phenotypes are reported. These are described in the following sections.

2.1.1 Haemophilia B Leyden

Haemophilia B Leyden is a specific type of HB in which the patient presents with decreased FIX:C levels in the early childhood, but the levels progressively increase after puberty. The disease is postulated to occur as a result of mutation in the 50 bp region that spans the transcriptional start site [25]. A total of 23 promoter region mutations have been identified until now (**Table 3**).

The mutation at c.-55G>C (or c. -26G>C in legacy nucleotide numbering) found in the promoter region of F9 gene is also called the haemophilia B Brandenburg mutation [38]. Unlike HB Leyden this variant does not exhibit improvement in FIX: C levels with age. The promoter region sequence located at c.-34 to -10 of the F9 gene serves as a binding site for the hepatocyte nuclear factor 4 (HNF4). The liver-enriched HNF4 is a member of the steroid hormone receptor superfamily of transcription factors (also called the nuclear receptor superfamily). Mutation at HNF4

HGVS cDNA name	Legacy nucleotide no.	Nature of mutation	Disease severity	Reference
c.-55G>A	-26	Substitution	Moderate	[26]
c.-55G>C	-26	Substitution	Severe	[27]
c.-55G>T	-26	Substitution	Severe	[28]
c.-53A>G	-24	Substitution	Not reported	[21]
c.-52C>G	-23	Substitution	Not reported	[21]
c.-52C>T	-23	Substitution	Not reported	[29]
c.-50T>G	-21	Substitution	Not reported	[30]
c.-49T>A	-20	Substitution	Moderate/mild	[31]
c.-49T>C	-20	Substitution	Mild	[32]
c.-48G>C	-19	Substitution	Moderate/mild	[29]
c.-35G>A	-6	Substitution	Mild	[33]
c.-35G>C	-6	Substitution	Mild	[34]
c.-34A>G	-5	Substitution	Mild	[26]
c.-34A>T	-5	Substitution	Moderate	[35]
c.-24T>A	6	Substitution	Mild	[34]
c.-23T>C	7	Substitution	Not reported	[21]
c.-22T>C/c	8	Substitution	Mild	[36]
c.-22delT	8	Deletion	Moderate	[21]
c.-21C>G	9	Substitution	Not reported	[21]
c.-18A>G	12	Substitution	Moderate	[21]
c.-17A>C	13	Substitution	Severe	[26]
c.-17A>G	13	Substitution	Mild	[37]
c.-17delA	13	Deletion	Mild	[37]

HGVS, Human Genome Variation Society; no., number.

Table 3.
F9 promoter site mutations associated with HB Leyden (mutation c.-55G>C is an exception).

disrupts the binding site to variable extents of severity. The mutation c.-55G>C, however, occurs at a site which is overlapped by the HNF4 binding site and another regulatory region, the androgen-responsive element (ARE) [39].

2.1.2 Thrombophilia

The F9 mutation c.1151G>T is associated with several fold increase in FIX:C activity [40]. The mutant FIX has leucine substituted for arginine at p.Arg384Leu. This alteration increases the affinity for FX to bind at this site. Patients might present with thromboembolic complications. This variant was named 'factor IX Padua'. Studies have also demonstrated that Arg-338 is part of an exosite (a secondary binding site) that binds factor X and heparin at the same time [41].

People with FIX:C levels more than 129 U/dL are 2–3 times more at risk of developing DVT in comparison to those with lower FIX:C levels. The risk is higher in females [42]. Variations in F9-associated single-nucleotide polymorphisms (SNPs) do not explain this raise in FIX antigen levels [43].

2.1.3 Protection against DVT

The Malmo polymorphism, c.580G>A (p. Ala194Thr), has an allele frequency of 0.32 in the Western population. It has been found that people with the G allele (F9 Malmo) have a 15–43% decreased risk of developing DVT in comparison to those with A allele [44]. This protective role of F9 Malmo has been extensively studied and confirmed [45]. The biochemical mechanisms behind this phenomenon are still obscure.

2.1.4 Warfarin sensitivity

All vitamin K-dependent clotting factors [including FII, FVII, FIX, FX, protein C (PC), protein S (PS) and protein Z (PZ)] possess an 18 amino acid propeptide sequence which serves as a binding site for the γ-glutamyl carboxylase enzyme. This enzyme catalyses modification of certain glutamate residues in the amino terminus of the mentioned clotting factors [46]. It has been determined that mutations at this site reduce the affinity vitamin K-dependent γ-carboxylase for the proteins.

3. Phenotypic plasticity

Phenotypic plasticity is defined as 'the ability of individual genotypes to produce different phenotypes when exposed to different environmental conditions' [47]. In the current scenario, this refers to presentation of the same mutation with different severities of the disease.

3.1 Genetic basis of phenotypic plasticity

It has been found that the mutations with varying phenotypes (MVPs) mostly occur at the less conserved sites with Arg being the usual mutated residue. It is also noted that these mutations commonly occur at the CpG dinucleotides. In comparison, mutations with uniform phenotypes (MUPs) occur in more conserved sites, with cysteine as the most frequently mutated amino acid residue. Intrinsic protein structural changes have been reported with reduced severity in cases of MVPs. No significant structural variations are identified between the two groups. The phenomenon is hypothesised to be a function of multiple factors including modifier

HGVS cDNA	HGVS protein	Mutation type	Mechanism	Exon	Domain	Severe (<1 U/dL)	Moderate (1–5 U/dL)	Mild (>5 U/dL)
c.1171C>T	p.Arg391Cys	Missense	Substitution	8	a1	X	X	X
c.1172G>A	p.Arg391His	Missense	Substitution	8	a1	X	X	X
c.1492G>A	p.Gly498Arg	Missense	Substitution	10	A2	X	X	X
c.396A>C	p.Glu132Asp	Missense	Substitution	4	A1	X	X	X
c.4380delT	p.Asn1460Lysfs*5	Frameshift	Deletion	14	B	X	X	X
c.5122C>T	p.Arg1708Cys	Missense	Substitution	14	a3	X	X	X
c.5219+3A>G		Splice site change	Substitution	Intron 14		X	X	X
c.5399G>A	p.Arg1800His	Missense	Substitution	16	A3	X	X	X
c.5663G>T	p.Arg1888Ile	Missense	Substitution	17	A3	X	X	X
c.590T>G	p.Val197Gly	Missense	Substitution	4	A1	X	X	X
c.6356A>G	p.Gln2119Arg	Missense	Substitution	22	C1	X	X	X
c.6371A>G	p.Tyr2124Cys	Missense	Substitution	22	C1	X	X	X
c.6506G>A	p.Arg2169His	Missense	Substitution	23	C1	X	X	X
c.6545G>A	p.Arg2182His	Missense	Substitution	23	C1	X	X	X
c.6683G>A	p.Arg2228Gln	Missense	Substitution	24	C2	X	X	X
c.6977G>A	p.Arg2326Gln	Missense	Substitution	26	C2	X	X	X
c.902G>A	p.Arg301His	Missense	Substitution	7	A1	X	X	X
c.1063C>T	p.Arg355*	Nonsense	Substitution	8	A1	X	X	
c.1226A>G	p.Glu409Gly	Missense	Substitution	8	A2	X	X	
c.1316G>T	p.Gly439Val	Missense	Substitution	9	A2	X	X	
c.143+1567A>G		Splice site change	Substitution	Intron 1		X	X	
c.1475A>G	p.Tyr492Cys	Missense	Substitution	10	A2	X	X	

DOI: http://dx.doi.org/10.5772/intechopen.81429

HGVS cDNA	HGVS protein	Mutation type	Mechanism	Exon	Domain	Severe (<1 U/dL)	Moderate (1–5 U/dL)	Mild (>5 U/dL)
c.1639T>C	p.Cys547Arg	Missense	Substitution	11	A2	X	X	
c.1702G>A	p.Gly568Ser	Missense	Substitution	11	A2	X	X	
c.1754T>C	p.Ile585Thr	Missense	Substitution	12	A2	X	X	
c.1804C>T	p.Arg602*	Nonsense	Substitution	12	A2	X	X	
c.1809C>G	p.Ser603Arg	Missense	Substitution	12	A2	X	X	
c.2015_2017del	p.Phe672del	Small structural change (in-frame, <50 bp)	Deletion	13	A2	X	X	
c.2048A>G	p.Tyr683Cys	Missense	Substitution	13	A2	X	X	
c.206_212del	p.Leu69Glnfs*21	Frameshift	Deletion	2	A1	X	X	
c.2090T>A	p.Val697Asp	Missense	Substitution	13	A2	X	X	
c.2114-?_5219+?del		Large structural change (>50 bp)	Deletion	14	A3	X	X	
c.2159G>A	p.Gly720Asp	Missense	Substitution	14	A2	X	X	
c.2182delT	p.Ser728Leufs*23	Frameshift	Deletion	14	A2	X	X	
c.2373G>A	p.Trp791*	Nonsense	Substitution	14	B	X	X	
c.2440C>T	p.Arg814*	Nonsense	Substitution	14	B	X	X	
c.266G>A	p.Gly89Asp	Missense	Substitution	3	A1	X	X	
c.2945dupA	p.Asn982Lysfs*9	Frameshift	Duplication	14	B	X	X	
c.296T>A	p.Val99Asp	Missense	Substitution	3	A1	X	X	
c.3143G>A	p.Trp1048*	Nonsense	Substitution	14	B	X	X	
c.3300dupA	p.Glu1101Argfs*17	Frameshift	Duplication	14	B	X	X	
c.353A>G	p.His118Arg	Missense	Substitution	3	A1	X	X	
c.3637delA	p.Ile1213Phefs*5	Frameshift	Deletion	14	B	X	X	
c.3637dupA	p.Ile1213Asnfs*28	Frameshift	Duplication	14	B	X	X	

HGVS cDNA	HGVS protein	Mutation type	Mechanism	Exon	Domain	Severe (<1 U/dL)	Moderate (1–5 U/dL)	Mild (>5 U/dL)
c.3702_3705del	p.His1234Glnfs*2	Frameshift	Deletion	14	B	X	X	
c.388G>C	p.Gly130Arg	Missense	Substitution	3	A1	X	X	
c.421G>A	p.Glu141Lys	Missense	Substitution	4	A1	X	X	
c.4296_4300del	p.His1434Serfs*6	Frameshift	Deletion	14	B	X	X	
c.4379dupA	p.Asn1460Lysfs*2	Frameshift	Duplication	14	B	X	X	
c.43C>T	p.Arg15*	Nonsense	Substitution	1	Signal	X	X	
c.4796G>A	p.Trp1599*	Nonsense	Substitution	14	B	X	X	
c.4825dupA	p.Thr1609Asnfs*4	Frameshift	Duplication	14	B	X	X	
c.491G>A	p.Gly164Asp	Missense	Substitution	4	A1	X	X	
c.5113C>T	p.Gln1705*	Nonsense	Substitution	14	a3	X	X	
c.515G>T	p.Cys172Phe	Missense	Substitution	4	A1	X	X	
c.5219G>T	p.Arg1740Met	Missense	Substitution	14	A3	X	X	
c.5471dupA	p.Asn1824Lysfs*6	Frameshift	Duplication	16	A3	X	X	
c.5536A>T	p.Lys1846*	Nonsense	Substitution	16	A3	X	X	
c.556G>T	p.Asp186Tyr	Missense	Substitution	4	A1	X	X	
c.5606G>T	p.Gly1869Val	Missense	Substitution	17	A3	X	X	
c.5685delT	p.Phe1895Leufs*50	Frameshift	Deletion	17	A3	X	X	
c.5719A>T	p.Ser1907Cys	Missense	Substitution	17	A3	X	X	
c.5878C>T	p.Arg1960*	Nonsense	Substitution	18	A3	X	X	
c.5953C>T	p.Arg1985*	Nonsense	Substitution	18	A3	X	X	
c.5973_5976del	p.Met1992Hisfs*37	Frameshift	Deletion	18	A3	X	X	
c.5998+1G>A		Splice site change	Substitution	Intron 18		X	X	

HGVS cDNA	HGVS protein	Mutation type	Mechanism	Exon	Domain	Severe (<1 U/dL)	Moderate (1–5 U/dL)	Mild (>5 U/dL)
c.5999-?_6429+?dup		Large structural change (>50 bp)	Duplication	19–22		X	X	
c.602-?_787+?del		Large structural change (>50 bp)	Deletion	5–6		X	X	
c.6046C>T	p.Arg2016Trp	Missense	Substitution	19	A3	X	X	
c.6133G>A	p.Gly2045Arg	Missense	Substitution	20	C1	X	X	
c.6172G>C	p.Ala2058Pro	Missense	Substitution	20	C1	X	X	
c.6274-?_6429+?del		Large structural change (>50 bp)	Deletion	22	C1	X	X	
c.6403C>T	p.Arg2135*	Nonsense	Substitution	22	C1	X	X	
c.6429+?_6430-?inv		Large structural change (>50 bp)	Inversion	Intron 22		X	X	
c.6481C>T	p.Pro2161Ser	Missense	Substitution	23	C1	X	X	
c.6485C>T	p.Pro2162Leu	Missense	Substitution	23	C1	X	X	
c.6496C>T	p.Arg2166*	Nonsense	Substitution	23	C1	X	X	
c.6544C>T	p.Arg2182Cys	Missense	Substitution	23	C1	X	X	
c.6593G>T	p.Gly2198Val	Missense	Substitution	24	C2	X	X	
c.6682C>G	p.Arg2228Gly	Missense	Substitution	24	C2	X	X	
c.6682C>T	p.Arg2228*	Nonsense	Substitution	24	C2	X	X	
c.670+5G>A		Splice site change	Substitution	Intron 5		X	X	
c.6742T>A	p.Trp2248Arg	Missense	Substitution	25	C2	X	X	
c.6875_6876del	p.Phe2294Serfs*90	Frameshift	Deletion	25	C2	X	X	
c.6967C>T	p.Arg2323Cys	Missense	Substitution	26	C2	X	X	
c.6977G>T	p.Arg2326Leu	Missense	Substitution	26	C2	X	X	
c.6994T>C	p.Trp2332Arg	Missense	Substitution	26	C2	X	X	
c.764G>C	p.Gly255Ala	Missense	Substitution	6	A1	X	X	

HGVS cDNA	HGVS protein	Mutation type	Mechanism	Exon	Domain	Severe (<1 U/dL)	Moderate (1–5 U/dL)	Mild (>5 U/dL)
c.785C>T	p.Pro262Leu	Missense	Substitution	6	A1	X	X	
c.787+3A>G		Splice site change	Substitution	Intron 6		X	X	
c.822G>C	p.Trp274Cys	Missense	Substitution	7	A1	X	X	
c.901C>T	p.Arg301Cys	Missense	Substitution	7	A1	X	X	
c.954_955del	p.Leu319Aspfs*18	Frameshift	Deletion	7	A1	X	X	
c.991_992del	p.Ile331Leufs*6	Frameshift	Deletion	7	A1	X	X	
c.1043G>A	p.Cys348Tyr	Missense	Substitution	8	A1	X		X
c.121G>T	p.Gly41Cys	Missense	Substitution	1	A1	X		X
c.1409C>T	p.Pro470Leu	Missense	Substitution	9	A2	X		X
c.1751A>G	p.Gln584Arg	Missense	Substitution	11	A2	X		X
c.1910A>G	p.Asn637Ser	Missense	Substitution	13	A2	X		X
c.3870dupA	p.Gly1291Argfs*29	Frameshift	Duplication	14	B	X		X
c.437A>C	p.Lys146Thr	Missense	Substitution	4	A1	X		X
c.5150A>G	p.Tyr1717Cys	Missense	Substitution	14	A3	X		X
c.5183A>G	p.Tyr1728Cys	Missense	Substitution	14	A3	X		X
c.6273+1G>T		Splice site change	Substitution	Intron 21		X		X
c.677G>T	p.Ser226Ile	Missense	Substitution	6	A1	X		X
c.6967C>G	p.Arg2323Gly	Missense	Substitution	26	C2	X		X
c.902G>T	p.Arg301Leu	Missense	Substitution	7	A1	X		X
c.923C>T	p.Ser308Leu	Missense	Substitution	7	A1	X		X
c.1293G>T	p.Leu431Phe	Missense	Substitution	9	A2		X	X
c.1348T>A	p.Tyr450Asn	Missense	Substitution	9	A2		X	X
c.1408C>A	p.Pro470Thr	Missense	Substitution	9	A2		X	X

HGVS cDNA	HGVS protein	Mutation type	Mechanism	Exon	Domain	Severe (<1 U/dL)	Moderate (1–5 U/dL)	Mild (>5 U/dL)
c.1569G>T	p.=	Synonymous	Substitution	11	A2		X	X
c.1636C>T	p.Arg546Trp	Missense	Substitution	11	A2		X	X
c.1648C>T	p.Arg550Cys	Missense	Substitution	11	A2		X	X
c.1660A>G	p.Ser554Gly	Missense	Substitution	11	A2		X	X
c.1834C>T	p.Arg612Cys	Missense	Substitution	12	A2		X	X
c.2044G>T	p.Val682Phe	Missense	Substitution	13	A2		X	X
c.2149C>T	p.Arg717Trp	Missense	Substitution	14	A2		X	X
c.2167G>A	p.Ala723Thr	Missense	Substitution	14	A2		X	X
c.274G>A	p.Gly92Ser	Missense	Substitution	3	A1		X	X
c.311T>A	p.Val104Asp	Missense	Substitution	3	A1		X	X
c.410C>T	p.Thr137Ile	Missense	Substitution	4	A1		X	X
c.5096A>T	p.Tyr1699Phe	Missense	Substitution	14	a3		X	X
c.5143C>G	p.Arg1715Gly	Missense	Substitution	14	A3		X	X
c.5339C>A	p.Pro1780Gln	Missense	Substitution	15	A3		X	X
c.5393C>T	p.Ala1798Val	Missense	Substitution	16	A3		X	X
c.5398C>G	p.Arg1800Gly	Missense	Substitution	16	A3		X	X
c.541G>A	p.Val181Met	Missense	Substitution	4	A1		X	X
c.5428T>C	p.Ser1810Pro	Missense	Substitution	16	A3		X	X
c.5526G>A	p.Met1842Ile	Missense	Substitution	16	A3		X	X
c.5557G>A	p.Ala1853Thr	Missense	Substitution	16	A3		X	X
c.5618C>T	p.Pro1873Leu	Missense	Substitution	17	A3		X	X
c.5825G>C	p.Gly1942Ala	Missense	Substitution	18	A3		X	X
c.5879G>A	p.Arg1960Gln	Missense	Substitution	18	A3		X	X

HGVS cDNA	HGVS protein	Mutation type	Mechanism	Exon	Domain	Severe (<1 U/dL)	Moderate (1–5 U/dL)	Mild (>5 U/dL)
c.5921C>T	p.Ser1974Phe	Missense	Substitution	18	A3		X	X
c.5954G>A	p.Arg1985Gln	Missense	Substitution	18	A3		X	X
c.601+1632G>A		Splice site change	Substitution	Intron 4			X	X
c.6113A>G	p.Asn2038Ser	Missense	Substitution	19	A3		X	X
c.6119G>A	p.Cys2040Tyr	Missense	Substitution	20	C1		X	X
c.6212G>C	p.Arg2071Thr	Missense	Substitution	21	C1		X	X
c.6278A>G	p.Asp2093Gly	Missense	Substitution	22	C1		X	X
c.6350T>G	p.Ile2117Ser	Missense	Substitution	22	C1		X	X
c.6413C>A	p.Ser2138Tyr	Missense	Substitution	22	C1		X	X
c.6443A>G	p.Asn2148Ser	Missense	Substitution	23	C1		X	X
c.6520C>G	p.His2174Asp	Missense	Substitution	23	C1		X	X
c.6532C>T	p.Arg2178Cys	Missense	Substitution	23	C1		X	X
c.668A>C	p.Glu223Ala	Missense	Substitution	5	A1		X	X
c.670+6T>C		Splice site change	Substitution	Intron 5			X	X
c.6744G>T	p.Trp2248Cys	Missense	Substitution	25	C2		X	X
c.67A>G	p.Arg23Gly	Missense	Substitution	1	A1		X	X
c.6915T>G	p.Asn2305Lys	Missense	Substitution	26	C2		X	X
c.6920A>C	p.Asp2307Ala	Missense	Substitution	26	C2		X	X
c.6956C>T	p.Pro2319Leu	Missense	Substitution	26	C2		X	X
c.755C>T	p.Thr252Ile	Missense	Substitution	6	A1		X	X
c.871G>A	p.Glu291Lys	Missense	Substitution	7	A1		X	X

Table 4.
List of F8 mutations reported with phenotypic plasticity.

HGVS cDNA name	HGVS protein name	Mutation type	Mechanism	Exon	Domain	Severe (< 1 U/dL)	Moderate (1–5 U/dL)	Mild (>5 U/dL)
c.87A>G	p.Thr29Thr	Synonymous	Substitution	1	PRO	X	X	X
c.127C>T	p.Arg43Trp	Missense	Substitution	2	PRO	X	X	X
c.128G>A	p.Arg43Gln	Missense	Substitution	2	PRO	X	X	X
c.172G>A	p.Gly58Arg	Missense	Substitution	2	GLA	X	X	X
c.173G>A	p.Gly58Glu	Missense	Substitution	2	GLA	X	X	X
c.191G>A	p.Cys64Tyr	Missense	Substitution	2	GLA	X	X	X
c.259T>G	p.Phe87Val	Missense	Substitution	3	GLA	X	X	X
c.301C>G	p.Pro101Ala	Missense	Substitution	4	EGF1	X	X	X
c.316G>A	p.Gly106Ser	Missense	Substitution	4	EGF1	X	X	X
c.412A>C	p.Asn138His	Missense	Substitution	5	EGF2	X	X	X
c.415G>A	p.Gly139Ser	Missense	Substitution	5	EGF2	X	X	X
c.571C>T	p.Arg191Cys	Missense	Substitution	6	Linker	X	X	X
c.572G>A	p.Arg191His	Missense	Substitution	6	Linker	X	X	X
c.720G>T	p.Trp240Cys	Missense	Substitution	6	Protease	X	X	X
c.755G>A	p.Cys252Tyr	Missense	Substitution	7	Protease	X	X	X
c.797C>T	p.Ala266Val	Missense	Substitution	7	Protease	X	X	X
c.835G>A	p.Ala279Thr	Missense	Substitution	7	Protease	X	X	X
c.838G>C	p.Gly280Arg	Missense	Substitution	7	Protease	X	X	X
c.881G>A	p.Arg294Gln	Missense	Substitution	8	Protease	X	X	X
c.914A>G	p.Tyr305Cys	Missense	Substitution	8	Protease	X	X	X
c.987C>G	p.Ser329Arg	Missense	Substitution	8	Protease	X	X	X
c.1009G>A	p.Ala337Thr	Missense	Substitution	8	Protease	X	X	X

HGVS cDNA name	HGVS protein name	Mutation type	Mechanism	Exon	Domain	Severe (< 1 U/dL)	Moderate (1–5 U/dL)	Mild (>5 U/dL)
c.1025C>T	p.Thr342Met	Missense	Substitution	8	Protease	X	X	X
c.1135C>T	p.Arg379*	Nonsense	Substitution	8	Protease	X	X	X
c.1136G>A	p.Arg379Gln	Missense	Substitution	8	Protease	X	X	X
c.1187G>C	p.Cys396Ser	Missense	Substitution	8	Protease	X	X	X
c.1235G>A	p.Gly412Glu	Missense	Substitution	8	Protease	X	X	X
c.1240C>A	p.Pro414Thr	Missense	Substitution	8	Protease	X	X	X
c.1275A>C	p.Leu425Phe	Missense	Substitution	8	Protease	X	X	X
c.1304G>A	p.Cys435Tyr	Missense	Substitution	8	Protease	X	X	X
c.1306G>A	p.Ala436Thr	Missense	Substitution	8	Protease	X	X	X
c.1328T>C	p.Ile443Thr	Missense	Substitution	8	Protease	X	X	X
c.*2545A>G		3′UTR	Substitution	3′UTR		X	X	X
c.-17A>G		Promoter	Substitution	1		X	X	X
c.-35G>A		Promoter	Substitution	5′UTR		X	X	X
c.-35G>C		Promoter	Substitution	5′UTR		X	X	X
c.50T>A	p.Ile17Asn	Missense	Substitution	1	Signal peptide	X	X	
c.83G>A	p.Cys28Tyr	Missense	Substitution	1	Signal peptide	X	X	
c.128G>T	p.Arg43Leu	Missense	Substitution	2	PRO	X	X	
c.138G>T	p.Arg47Ser	Missense	Substitution	2	PRO	X	X	
c.190T>C	p.Cys64Arg	Missense	Substitution	2	GLA	X	X	
c.199G>A	p.Glu67Lys	Missense	Substitution	2	GLA	X	X	
c.219A>C	p.Glu73Asp	Missense	Substitution	2	GLA	X	X	
c.223C>T	p.Arg75Stop	Nonsense	Substitution	2	GLA	X	X	

DOI: http://dx.doi.org/10.5772/intechopen.81429

HGVS cDNA name	HGVS protein name	Mutation type	Mechanism	Exon	Domain	Severe (< 1 U/dL)	Moderate (1–5 U/dL)	Mild (>5 U/dL)
c.226G>A	p.Glu76Lys	Missense	Substitution	2	GLA	X	X	
c.260T>G	p.Phe87Cys	Missense	Substitution	3	GLA	X	X	
c.263G>A	p.Trp88*	Nonsense	Substitution	3	GLA	X	X	
c.291T>G	p.Cys97Trp	Missense	Substitution	4	EGF1	X	X	
c.304T>C	p.Cys102Arg	Missense	Substitution	4	EGF1	X	X	
c.305G>A	p.Cys102Tyr	Missense	Substitution	4	EGF1	X	X	
c.350G>A	p.Cys117Tyr	Missense	Substitution	4	EGF1	X	X	
c.383G>A	p.Cys128Tyr	Missense	Substitution	4	EGF1	X	X	
c.392delA	p.Asp131fs	Frameshift	Deletion	5	EGF2	X	X	
c.414T>A	p.Asn138Lys	Missense	Substitution	5	EGF2	X	X	
c.422G>A	p.Cys141Tyr	Missense	Substitution	5	EGF2	X	X	
c.423C>A	p.Cys141*	Nonsense	Substitution	5	EGF2	X	X	
c.423C>G	p.Cys141Trp	Missense	Substitution	5	EGF2	X	X	
c.427C>G	p.Gln143Glu	Missense	Substitution	5	EGF2	X	X	
c.434G>A	p.Cys145Tyr	Missense	Substitution	5	EGF2	X	X	
c.464G>T	p.Cys155Phe	Missense	Substitution	5	EGF2	X	X	
c.470G>A	p.Cys157Tyr	Missense	Substitution	5	EGF2	X	X	
c.470G>C	p.Cys157Ser	Missense	Substitution	5	EGF2	X	X	
c.479G>T	p.Gly160Val	Missense	Substitution	5	EGF2	X	X	
c.482A>G	p.Tyr161Cys	Missense	Substitution	5	EGF2	X	X	
c.484C>T	p.Arg162*	Nonsense	Substitution	5	EGF2	X	X	
c.509G>A	p.Ser170Tyr	Missense	Substitution	5	EGF2	X	X	

HGVS cDNA name	HGVS protein name	Mutation type	Mechanism	Exon	Domain	Severe (< 1 U/dL)	Moderate (1–5 U/dL)	Mild (>5 U/dL)
c.520G>A	p.Val174Met	Missense	Substitution	5	EGF2	X	X	
c.532T>C	p.Cys178Arg	Missense	Substitution	6	Linker	X	X	
c.535G>A	p.Gly179Arg	Missense	Substitution	6	Linker	X	X	
c.545_546del	p.Ser182Cysfs*6	Frameshift	Deletion	6	Linker	X	X	
c.547delG	p.Val183fs	Frameshift	Deletion	6	Linker	X	X	
c.676C>T	p.Arg226Trp	Missense	Substitution	6	Activation	X	X	
c.677G>A	p.Arg226Gln	Missense	Substitution	6	Activation	X	X	
c.677G>T	p.Arg226Leu	Missense	Substitution	6	Activation	X	X	
c.688_690del	p.Gly230del	Small structural change (in-frame, <50 bp)	Deletion	6	Protease	X	X	
c.706G>T	p.Gly236Cys	Missense	Substitution	6	Protease	X	X	
c.707G>A	p.Gly236Asp	Missense	Substitution	6	Protease	X	X	
c.711A>G	p.Gln237Gln	Synonymous	Substitution	6	Protease	X	X	
c.719G>A	p.Trp240*	Nonsense	Substitution	6	Protease	X	X	
c.719G>T	p.Trp240Leu	Missense	Substitution	6	Protease	X	X	
c.721C>T	p.Gln241*	Nonsense	Substitution	6	Protease	X	X	
c.723G>A	p.Gln241Gln	Synonymous	Substitution	6	Protease	X	X	
c.727_728delinsA	p.Val243fs	Frameshift	Insertion/ deletion	7	Protease	X	X	
c.757G>A	p.Gly253Arg	Missense	Substitution	7	Protease	X	X	
c.789_790InsT	p.Thr264fs	Frameshift	Insertion	7	Protease	X	X	
c.799C>T	p.His267Tyr	Missense	Substitution	7	Protease	X	X	
c.839G>T	p.Gly280Val	Missense	Substitution	8	Protease	X	X	

HGVS cDNA name	HGVS protein name	Mutation type	Mechanism	Exon	Domain	Severe (< 1 U/dL)	Moderate (1–5 U/dL)	Mild (>5 U/dL)
c.871G>A	p.Glu291Lys	Missense	Substitution	8	Protease	X	X	
c.880C>T	p.Arg294*	Nonsense	Substitution	8	Protease	X	X	
c.881G>T	p.Arg294Leu	Missense	Substitution	8	Protease	X	X	
c.892C>T	p.Arg298*	Nonsense	Substitution	8	Protease	X	X	
c.946A>T	p.Ile316Phe	Missense	Substitution	8	Protease	X	X	
c.990C>A	p.Tyr330*	Nonsense	Substitution	8	Protease	X	X	
c.1004G>T	p.Cys335Tyr	Missense	Substitution	8	Protease	X	X	
c.1009G>C	p.Ala337Pro	Missense	Substitution	8	Protease	X	X	
c.1068G>C	p.Trp356Cys	Missense	Substitution	8	Protease	X	X	
c.1069G>A	p.Gly357Arg	Missense	Substitution	8	Protease	X	X	
c.1070G>A	p.Gly357Glu	Missense	Substitution	8	Protease	X	X	
c.1076T>G	p.Val359Gly	Missense	Substitution	8	Protease	X	X	
c.1097C>A	p.Ala366Asp	Missense	Substitution	8	Protease	X	X	
c.1108C>T	p.Gln370*	Nonsense	Substitution	8	Protease	X	X	
c.1113C>A	p.Tyr371*	Nonsense	Substitution	8	Protease	X	X	
c.1120G>T	p.Val374Glu	Missense	Substitution	8	Protease	X	X	
c.1135C>G	p.Arg379Gly	Missense	Substitution	8	Protease	X	X	
c.1144T>C	p.Cys382Arg	Missense	Substitution	8	Protease	X	X	
c.1147C>T	p.Leu383Phe	Missense	Substitution	8	Protease	X	X	
c.1150C>T	p.Arg384*	Nonsense	Substitution	8	Protease	X	X	
c.1168A>T	p.Ile390Phe	Missense	Substitution	8	Protease	X	X	
c.1169T>G	p.Ile390Ser	Missense	Substitution	8	Protease	X	X	

HGVS cDNA name	HGVS protein name	Mutation type	Mechanism	Exon	Domain	Severe (< 1 U/dL)	Moderate (1–5 U/dL)	Mild (>5 U/dL)
c.1181T>A	p.Met394Lys	Missense	Substitution	8	Protease	X	X	
c.1204G>A	p.Gly402Arg	Missense	Substitution	8	Protease	X	X	
c.1217C>G	p.Ser406*	Nonsense	Substitution	8	Protease	X	X	
c.1217C>T	p.Ser406Leu	Missense	Substitution	8	Protease	X	X	
c.1219T>C	p.Cys407Arg	Missense	Substitution	8	Protease	X	X	
c.1226G>A	p.Gly409Glu	Missense	Substitution	8	Protease	X	X	
c.1228G>A	p.Asp410Asn	Missense	Substitution	8	Protease	X	X	
c.1228G>C	p.Asp410His	Missense	Substitution	8	Protease	X	X	
c.1232G>A	p.Ser411Asn	Missense	Substitution	8	Protease	X	X	
c.1237G>A	p.Gly413Arg	Missense	Substitution	8	Protease	X	X	
c.1241C>T	p.Pro414Leu	Missense	Substitution	8	Protease	X	X	
c.1245T>A	p.His415Gln	Missense	Substitution	8	Protease	X	X	
c.1256T>A	p.Val419Glu	Missense	Substitution	8	Protease	X	X	
c.1258G>T	p.Glu420*	Nonsense	Substitution	8	Protease	X	X	
c.1291T>C	p.Trp431Arg	Missense	Substitution	8	Protease	X	X	
c.1293G>T	p.Trp431Cys	Missense	Substitution	8	Protease	X	X	
c.1294G>A	p.Gly432Ser	Missense	Substitution	8	Protease	X	X	
c.1295G>A	p.Gly432Asp	Missense	Substitution	8	Protease	X	X	
c.1295G>C	p.Gly432Ala	Missense	Substitution	8	Protease	X	X	
c.1295G>T	p.Gly432Val	Missense	Substitution	8	Protease	X	X	
c.1297G>A	p.Glu433Lys	Missense	Substitution	8	Protease	X	X	
c.1298A>C	p.Glu433Ala	Missense	Substitution	8	Protease	X	X	

HGVS cDNA name	HGVS protein name	Mutation type	Mechanism	Exon	Domain	Severe (< 1 U/dL)	Moderate (1–5 U/dL)	Mild (>5 U/dL)
c.1307C>T	p.Ala436Val	Missense	Substitution	8	Protease	X	X	
c.1318A>G	p.Lys440Glu	Missense	Substitution	8	Protease	X	X	
c.1324G>A	p.Gly442Arg	Missense	Substitution	8	Protease	X	X	
c.1357T>C	p.Trp453Arg	Missense	Substitution	8	Protease	X	X	
c.1361T>C	p.Ile454Thr	Missense	Substitution	8	Protease	X	X	
c.*1157A>G		3′UTR	Substitution	3′UTR		X	X	
c.252+3_252+6del		Splice site change	Deletion	Intron 2		X	X	
c.252+6T>C		Splice site change	Substitution	Intron 2		X	X	
c.253-25A>G		Splice site change	Substitution	Intron 2		X	X	
c.277+2T>C		Splice site change	Substitution	Intron 3		X	X	
c.277+5G>A		Splice site change	Substitution	Intron 3		X	X	
c.392-1G>C		Splice site change	Substitution	Intron 4		X	X	
c.392-2A>G		Splice site change	Substitution	Intron 4		X	X	
c.521-3T>G		Splice site change	Substitution	Intron 5		X	X	
c.-55G>A		Promoter	Substitution	5′UTR		X	X	
c.723+1G>A		Splice site change	Substitution	Intron 6		X	X	
c.839-4A>G		Splice site change	Substitution	Intron 7		X	X	
c.88+1_88+4del		Splice site change	Deletion	Intron 1		X	X	
c.88+1G>T		Splice site change	Substitution	Intron 1		X	X	
c.88+5G>C		Splice site change	Substitution	Intron 1		X	X	
c.88+5G>T		Splice site change	Substitution	Intron 1		X	X	
c.19A>T	p.Ile7Phe	Missense	Substitution	1	Signal peptide	X		X

HGVS cDNA name	HGVS protein name	Mutation type	Mechanism	Exon	Domain	Severe (< 1 U/dL)	Moderate (1–5 U/dL)	Mild (>5 U/dL)
c.164T>G	p.Phe55Cys	Missense	Substitution	2	GLA	X		X
c.339T>A	p.Asn113Lys	Missense	Substitution	4	EGF1	X		X
c.466T>C	p.Ser156Phe	Missense	Substitution	5	EGF2	X		X
c.676C>G	p.Arg226Gly	Missense	Substitution	6	Activation	X		X
c.685G>A	p.Gly229Ser	Missense	Substitution	6	Protease	X		X
c.907C>T	p.His303Tyr	Missense	Substitution	8	Protease	X		X
c.942T>G	p.His314Gln	Missense	Substitution	8	Protease	X		X
c.1045G>T	p.Gly349*	Nonsense	Substitution	8	Protease	X		X
c.1072A>G	p.Arg358Gly	Missense	Substitution	8	Protease	X		X
c.1079T>C	p.Phe360Ser	Missense	Substitution	8	Protease	X		X
c.1109A>C	p.Gln370Pro	Missense	Substitution	8	Protease	X		X
c.1174A>G	p.Asn392Asp	Missense	Substitution	8	Protease	X		X
c.1238G>A	p.Gly413Glu	Missense	Substitution	8	Protease	X		X
c.252+5G>A		Splice site change	Substitution	Intron 2		X		X
c.839-1G>A		Splice site change	Substitution	Intron 7		X		X
c.82T>C	p.Cys28Arg	Missense	Substitution	1	Signal peptide		X	X
c.151A>G	p.Lys51Glu	Missense	Substitution	2	GLA		X	X
c.163T>A	p.Phe55Ile	Missense	Substitution	2	GLA		X	X
c.279T>A	p.Asp93Glu	Missense	Substitution	4	EGF1		X	X
c.335T>C	p.Ile112Thr	Missense	Substitution	4	EGF1		X	X
c.479G>A	p.Gly160Glu	Missense	Substitution	5	EGF2		X	X
c.479G>C	p.Gly160Ala	Missense	Substitution	5	EGF2		X	X

HGVS cDNA name	HGVS protein name	Mutation type	Mechanism	Exon	Domain	Severe (< 1 U/dL)	Moderate (1–5 U/dL)	Mild (>5 U/dL)
c.484C>A	p.Arg162Arg	Synonymous	Substitution	5	EGF2		X	X
c.572G>C	p.Arg191Pro	Missense	Substitution	6	Linker		X	X
c.785T>C	p.Ile262Thr	Missense	Substitution	7	Protease		X	X
c.786T>G	p.Ile262Met	Missense	Substitution	7	Protease		X	X
c.839G>C	p.Gly280Ala	Missense	Substitution	8	Protease		X	X
c.872A>G	p.Glu291Gly	Missense	Substitution	8	Protease		X	X
c.950C>T	p.Ala317Val	Missense	Substitution	8	Protease		X	X
c.997C>A	p.Pro333Thr	Missense	Substitution	8	Protease		X	X
c.1067G>T	p.Trp356Leu	Missense	Substitution	8	Protease		X	X
c.1097C>T	p.Ala366Val	Missense	Substitution	8	Protease		X	X
c.1127T>C	p.Leu376Pro	Missense	Substitution	8	Protease		X	X
c.1180A>G	p.Met394Val	Missense	Substitution	8	Protease		X	X
c.1187G>T	p.Cys396Phe	Missense	Substitution	8	Protease		X	X
c.1193G>C	p.Gly398Ala	Missense	Substitution	8	Protease		X	X
c.1348T>C	p.Tyr450His	Missense	Substitution	8	Protease		X	X
c.-48G>C		Promoter	Substitution	5′UTR			X	X
c.-49T>A		Promoter	Substitution	5′UTR			X	X
c.520+13A>G		Splice site change	Substitution	Intron 5			X	X
c.88+5G>A		Splice site change	Substitution	Intron 1			X	X

Table 5.
List of F9 mutations reported with phenotypic plasticity.

genes, epigenetic influences and environmental effects. These factors may act individually or in combination [48].

Tables 4 and **5** depict F8 and F9 mutations, respectively, reported with phenotypic plasticity [49, 50]. A total of 351 mutations are presented here with cases reported from at least two severity classes. The most significant are the 85 cases (32 from F8 and 53 from F9) wherein patients from both severe and mild categories are reported.

Taking into account the significant amount of phenotypic plasticity in haemophilia, researchers have proposed to recognise the disease phenotype, in terms of coagulation activity, a continuous variable and abandoning of the classical categorical classification [51]. With the evolving concepts of personalised medicine, this may prove realistic... and the future.

Author details

Muhammad Tariq Masood Khan[1]* and Abid Sohail Taj[2]

1 Northwest School of Medicine, Peshawar, Pakistan

2 Peshawar General Hospital, Peshawar, Pakistan

*Address all correspondence to: drtariqmsd@gmail.com

IntechOpen

© 2019 The Author(s). Licensee IntechOpen. This chapter is distributed under the terms of the Creative Commons Attribution License (http://creativecommons.org/licenses/by/3.0), which permits unrestricted use, distribution, and reproduction in any medium, provided the original work is properly cited.

References

[1] Jayandharan GR, Srivastava A. The phenotypic heterogeneity of severe hemophilia. Seminars in Thrombosis and Hemostasis. 2008;**34**(1):128-141

[2] Wojczynski MK, Tiwari HK. Definition of phenotype. Advances in Genetics. 2008;**60**:75-105

[3] Schulze TG, McMahon FJ. Defining the phenotype in human genetic studies: Forward genetics and reverse phenotyping. Human Heredity. 2004;**58** (3–4):131-138

[4] Winawer MR. Phenotype definition in epilepsy. Epilepsy & Behavior: E&B. 2006;**8**(3):462-476

[5] Gottesman II, Gould TD. The endophenotype concept in psychiatry: Etymology and strategic intentions. The American Journal of Psychiatry. 2003; **160**(4):636-645

[6] Schramm W. The history of haemophilia—A short review. Thrombosis Research. 2014;**134** (Supp. 1):S4-S9

[7] Ingram GI. The history of haemophilia. Journal of Clinical Pathology. 1976;**29**(6):469-479

[8] Franchini M, Mannucci PM. Past, present and future of hemophilia: A narrative review. Orphanet Journal of Rare Diseases. 2012;7:24

[9] White GC 2nd, Rosendaal F, Aledort LM, Lusher JM, Rothschild C, Ingerslev J. Definitions in hemophilia. Recommendation of the scientific subcommittee on factor VIII and factor IX of the scientific and standardization committee of the International Society on Thrombosis and Haemostasis. Thrombosis and Haemostasis. 2001;**85**(3):560

[10] Konkle BA, Josephson NC, Nakaya Fletcher S. Hemophilia B. In: GeneReviews®. Seattle, WA: University of Washington, Seattle. 2000. Available from: https://www.ncbi.nlm.nih.gov/books/NBK1495/

[11] Konkle BA, Huston H, Nakaya Fletcher S. Hemophilia A. In: Adam MP, Ardinger HH, Pagon RA, Wallace SE, LJH B, Stephens K, et al., editors. GeneReviews((R)). Seattle (WA): University of Washington, Seattle; 1993. GeneReviews is a registered trademark of the University of Washington, Seattle. All rights reserved

[12] van den Berg HM, De Groot PH, Fischer K. Phenotypic heterogeneity in severe hemophilia. Journal of Thrombosis and Haemostasis. 2007;**5** (Supp. 1):151-156

[13] Khan MTM, Naz A, Ahmed J, Shamsi T, Ahmed S, Ahmed N, et al. Mutation spectrum and genotype-phenotype analyses in a Pakistani cohort with hemophilia B. Clinical and Applied Thrombosis/Hemostasis: Official Journal of the International Academy of Clinical and Applied Thrombosis/Hemostasis. 2018;**24**(5):741-748

[14] Zhao H, Yang Y, Lu Y, Mort M, Cooper DN, Zuo Z, et al. Quantitative mapping of genetic similarity in human heritable diseases by shared mutations. Human Mutation. 2018; **39**(2):292-301

[15] Graw J, Brackmann HH, Oldenburg J, Schramm W, Schwaab R, editors. Genotype-phenotype correlation in hemophilia A. In: 30th Hemophilia Symposium Hamburg 1999; Berlin/Heidelberg: Springer; 2001

[16] Zlotogora J. Penetrance and expressivity in the molecular age. Genetics in Medicine: Official Journal of the American College of Medical Genetics. 2003;**5**(5):347-352

[17] Pavlova A, Oldenburg J. Defining severity of hemophilia: More than factor levels. Seminars in Thrombosis and Hemostasis. 2013;**39**(7):702-710

[18] Baye TM, Abebe T, Wilke RA. Genotype-environment interactions and their translational implications. Personalized Medicine. 2011;**8**(1):59-70

[19] Chanda P, Sucheston L, Liu S, Zhang A, Ramanathan M. Information-theoretic gene-gene and gene-environment interaction analysis of quantitative traits. BMC Genomics. 2009;**10**:509

[20] Guo SW. Gene-environment interaction and the mapping of complex traits: Some statistical models and their implications. Human Heredity. 2000; **50**(5):286-303

[21] Rallapalli PM, Kemball-Cook G, Tuddenham EG, Gomez K, Perkins SJ. An interactive mutation database for human coagulation factor IX provides novel insights into the phenotypes and genetics of hemophilia B. Journal of Thrombosis and Haemostasis. 2013; **11**(7):1329-1340

[22] Plug I, Mauser-Bunschoten EP, Brocker-Vriends AH, van Amstel HK, van der Bom JG, van Diemen-Homan JE, et al. Bleeding in carriers of hemophilia. Blood. 2006;**108**(1):52-56

[23] Paroskie A, Gailani D, DeBaun MR, Sidonio RF Jr. A cross-sectional study of bleeding phenotype in haemophilia A carriers. British Journal of Haematology. 2015;**170**(2):223-228

[24] Khan MTM, Naz A, Ahmed J, Shamsi TS, Taj AS. Diagnosis and phenotypic assessment of Pakistani haemophilia B carriers. Pakistan Journal of Medical Sciences. 2017;**33**(3):738-742

[25] Picketts DJ, Lillicrap DP, Mueller CR. Synergy between transcription factors DBP and C/EBP compensates for a haemophilia B Leyden factor IX mutation. Nature Genetics. 1993;**3**(2): 175-179

[26] Giannelli F, Green PM, Sommer SS, Poon MC, Ludwig M, Schwaab R, et al. Haemophilia B (sixth edition): A database of point mutations and short additions and deletions. Nucleic Acids Research. 1996;**24**(1):103-118

[27] Crossley M, Winship PR, Austen DE, Rizza CR, Brownlee GG. A less severe form of haemophilia B Leyden. Nucleic Acids Research. 1990;**18**(15): 4633

[28] Belvini D, Salviato R, Radossi P, Pierobon F, Mori P, Castaldo G, et al. Molecular genotyping of the Italian cohort of patients with hemophilia B. Haematologica. 2005;**90**(5):635-642

[29] Ketterling RP, Liu JZ, Liao D, Kasper CK, Ambriz R, Paredes R, et al. Two novel factor IX promoter mutations: Incremental progress towards 'saturation in vivo mutagenesis' of a human promoter region. Human Molecular Genetics. 1995;**4**(4):769-770

[30] Reijnen MJ, Peerlinck K, Maasdam D, Bertina RM, Reitsma PH. Hemophilia B Leyden: Substitution of thymine for guanine at position −21 results in a disruption of a hepatocyte nuclear factor 4 binding site in the factor IX promoter. Blood. 1993;**82**(1):151-158

[31] Reitsma PH, Bertina RM, Ploos van Amstel JK, Riemens A, Briet E. The putative factor IX gene promoter in hemophilia B Leyden. Blood. 1988; **72**(3):1074-1076

[32] Ghanem N, Costes B, Martin J, Vidaud M, Rothschild C, Foyer-Gazengel C, et al. Twenty-four novel hemophilia B mutations revealed by rapid scanning of the whole factor IX gene in a French population sample. European Journal of Human Genetics. 1993;**1**(2):144-155

[33] Hirosawa S, Fahner JB, Salier JP, Wu CT, Lovrien EW, Kurachi K. Structural and functional basis of the developmental regulation of human coagulation factor IX gene: Factor IX Leyden. Proceedings of the National Academy of Sciences of the United States of America. 1990;**87**(12):4421-4425

[34] Stenson PD, Mort M, Ball EV, Howells K, Phillips AD, Thomas NS, et al. The human gene mutation database: 2008 update. Genome Medicine. 2009;**1**(1):13

[35] Picketts DJ, D'Souza C, Bridge PJ, Lillicrap D. An A to T transversion at position −5 of the factor IX promoter results in hemophilia B. Genomics. 1992; **12**(1):161-163

[36] Royle G, Van de Water NS, Berry E, Ockelford PA, Browett PJ. Haemophilia B Leyden arising de novo by point mutation in the putative factor IX promoter region. British Journal of Haematology. 1991;**77**(2):191-194

[37] Reitsma PH, Mandalaki T, Kasper CK, Bertina RM, Briet E. Two novel point mutations correlate with an altered developmental expression of blood coagulation factor IX (hemophilia B Leyden phenotype). Blood. 1989; **73**(3):743-746

[38] Bowen DJ. Haemophilia A and haemophilia B: Molecular insights. Molecular Pathology. 2002;**55**(1):1-18

[39] Crossley M, Ludwig M, Stowell KM, De Vos P, Olek K, Brownlee GG. Recovery from hemophilia B Leyden: An androgen-responsive element in the factor IX promoter. Science. 1992; **257**(5068):377-379

[40] Simioni P, Tormene D, Tognin G, Gavasso S, Bulato C, Iacobelli NP, et al. X-linked thrombophilia with a mutant factor IX (factor IX Padua). The New England Journal of Medicine. 2009; **361**(17):1671-1675

[41] Chang J, Jin J, Lollar P, Bode W, Brandstetter H, Hamaguchi N, et al. Changing residue 338 in human factor IX from arginine to alanine causes an increase in catalytic activity. The Journal of Biological Chemistry. 1998;**273**(20): 12089-12094

[42] van Hylckama Vlieg A, van der Linden IK, Bertina RM, Rosendaal FR. High levels of factor IX increase the risk of venous thrombosis. Blood. 2000; **95**(12):3678-3682

[43] van Minkelen R, de Visser MC, van Hylckama Vlieg A, Vos HL, Bertina RM. Sequence variants and haplotypes of the factor IX gene and the risk of venous thrombosis. Journal of Thrombosis and Haemostasis. 2008;**6**(9):1610-1613

[44] Bezemer ID, Bare LA, Doggen CJ, Arellano AR, Tong C, Rowland CM, et al. Gene variants associated with deep vein thrombosis. JAMA. 2008;**299**(11): 1306-1314

[45] Bezemer ID, Arellano AR, Tong CH, Rowland CM, Ireland HA, Bauer KA, et al. F9 Malmo, factor IX and deep vein thrombosis. Haematologica. 2009; **94**(5):693-699

[46] Stanley TB, Jin DY, Lin PJ, Stafford DW. The propeptides of the vitamin K-dependent proteins possess different affinities for the vitamin K-dependent carboxylase. The Journal of Biological Chemistry. 1999;**274**(24):16940-16944

[47] Fusco G, Minelli A. Phenotypic plasticity in development and evolution: Facts and concepts. Philosophical Transactions of the Royal Society, B: Biological Sciences. 2010;**365**(1540): 547-556

[48] Chavali S, Sharma A, Tabassum R, Bharadwaj D. Sequence and structural properties of identical mutations with varying phenotypes in human coagulation factor IX. Proteins. 2008; **73**(1):63-71

[49] Li T, Miller CH, Payne AB, Craig Hooper W. The CDC hemophilia B mutation project mutation list: A new online resource. Molecular Genetics & Genomic Medicine. 2013;**1**(4):238-245

[50] Payne AB, Miller CH, Kelly FM, Michael Soucie J, Craig Hooper W. The CDC hemophilia A mutation project (CHAMP) mutation list: A new online resource. Human Mutation. 2013;**34**(2): E2382-E2391

[51] Chavali S, Ghosh S, Bharadwaj D. Hemophilia B is a quasi-quantitative condition with certain mutations showing phenotypic plasticity. Genomics. 2009;**94**(6):433-437

Chapter 3

Perioperative Management of Hemophilia A Using Recombinant Factor VIII in Patients Undergoing Major or Minor Surgery

Atsushi Okamoto, Kenta Yamamoto, Go Eguchi, Yoshitaka Kanai, Terufumi Yamaguchi and Yasuhiro Maeda

Abstract

Among the surgical treatments performed in patients with hemophilia, joint surgery for intra-articular bleeding is the most time-consuming. Previous reports describe the perioperative management of hemophiliacs undergoing coronary artery bypass grafting or of those undergoing cystectomy for treatment of hematuria. In the former study, the patient was elderly; in the latter study, the authors concluded that cystectomy in hemophiliacs is safe if monitored appropriately and that urinary diversion using the intestine should be avoided because anastomotic hemorrhaging may occur. In this study, we discuss coagulation factor replacement therapy for patient with hemophilia A undergoing major or minor surgery.

Keywords: hemophilia, hemophilia with inhibitors, perioperative management, joint surgery

1. Introduction

Due to advancements in coagulation factor preparations, hemophilia treatment has progressed from conventional bleeding replacement therapy to periodic replacement therapy. Historically, the aim has been to perform symptomatic treatment, but currently, the aim of treatment is preventive. Due to bleeding incidents that are characteristic of hemophilia, control of bleeding is particularly important for perioperative patient management. The indication for surgical treatment in patients with hemophilia includes diseases caused by bleeding related to hemophilia as well as those not related to hemophilia. The number of surgeries involving patients with hemophilia is increasing annually.

Due to the development of hemostatic hemostasis treatments, obstacles due to bleeding in young patients are decreasing. However, surgical cases are increasing due to the trend in applying surgery to disorders, which have conventionally been treated nonsurgically and due to an increase in the number of aging patients as a result of improved life expectancy. Due to the reasons stated above, we consider that it is important to stay informed about the latest developments in the perioperative management of patients with hemophilia.

2. Preoperative preparation

Preoperative preparation for hemophiliac patients involves a thorough review of various aspects of the patient's condition. The first parameter to be ascertained is whether the hemophilia is of type A or type B. Following this, the severity of hemophilia needs to be confirmed. Hemophilia is classified based on the blood level of coagulation factors such as factor VIII or factor IX; the disease is characterized as severe when the blood coagulation factor level is less than 1%, moderate if it is 1–5%, and mild if the level is 5% or more. Severity of daily symptoms is generally accepted to reflect the severity of the disease. In patients receiving prophylactic replacement therapy, it is usually necessary to confirm details such as how many units are being administered and how the preparation is being self-injected. The presence of inhibitors (alloantibodies) in the blood needs to be checked as part of the preoperative preparation as well. Although it is known that patients with severe hemophilia are more likely to have developed inhibitors, genetic mutations are known to cause inhibitor formation even in cases with mild disease. Among patients who have received prior treatment, it is also important to check for HCV or HIV infections. Furthermore, if a chronic HCV infection is incident, liver cirrhosis or liver cancer may occur concomitantly, and it is thus necessary to screen patients for these conditions. The abovementioned points may be used as a checklist to evaluate the suitability of patients for surgical procedures. If the abovementioned evaluations reveal no issues, surgery may be performed as per usual protocol. Depending on the magnitude of the surgical invasion, a treatment plan may then be set up, detailing the target levels and of coagulation factors to be maintained, and the duration for which the levels need to be maintained. Regarding treatment planning, it is necessary to administer a necessary and sufficient amount of a coagulation factor preparation to prevent hemorrhagic complications. However, it should also be noted that an overdose of coagulation factor preparations can lead to a risk of thrombosis. The clearance of the coagulation factor preparation varies greatly among patients. In view of this fact, a pharmacokinetic test of factor VIII factor/factor IX preparations ideally to be used for surgery may be conducted preoperatively. Accurate pharmacokinetic profiles may be obtained by measuring coagulation factor activity before administration of the preparation, and 15 minutes, 1, 2, 4, 8, 12, and 24 hours after administration; such an evaluation allows for a proper understanding of the recovery rate and the half-life of the administered factors [1].

3. Selection of coagulation factor replenishment method

There are two main methods of administration of coagulation factor replacement therapy during surgery. The first method is a bolus administration method (BI method), which involves repeated administration of a bolus injections. The second is the continuous administration method (CI method) in which a syringe pump continuously administers coagulation factors after an initial bolus administration. Historically, the stability of the formulations used for coagulation factors has been poor; such formulations needed to be administered as soon as they were thawed. Therefore, perioperative management was predominantly performed using the BI method. In the BI method, when the coagulation factor is injected, the coagulation factor level in the blood exceeds 100% and gradually falls thereafter; when the level approaches 50%, the next bolus is administered. Bolus administration is repeated each time the blood coagulation factor level approaches 50%. The BI method has the advantage of being simple, although the associated disadvantage is that fluctuation in the coagulation factor levels is high. Intraoperative and postoperative bleeding in recurrent invasive surgery and reoperation is also a serious issue. Recently, however, the stability of the drug and the reliability of the syringe pump have been improved significantly, and the CI method is currently the recommended method for use during major surgery. Using the CI method, the blood clotting ability of hemophilia patients without inhibitors may be restored to that of non-hemophiliac subjects, so that the indication for surgery can be adjusted to the same level as that for non-hemophiliac subjects. Scientific evidence for the effectiveness of the CI method has been accumulating, and there are many reports of surgical cases in which the CI method has been used. However, because the CI method requires specialized expertise, it is desirable to conduct this procedure under the guidance of a hemophilia specialist. The BI and the CI methods have distinct advantages and disadvantages. For routine surgical operations predicted to have less bleeding volume, selection of the BI method according to the situation of the clinical site is appropriate. There have been few systematic studies of the BI method, and hence it cannot be officially recommended. However, as mentioned above, this method has historically been used extensively for numerous types of surgical procedures. The most important advantage of the BI method is that it is a simple method. Application of this method in emergency situations should be decided based on the trough value of the coagulation factor concentration in the blood or when there is insufficient preparation time and insufficient experience with the CI method. If the staff is experienced in performing the CI method, this method may be applied in emergency situations; a provisional administration speed may be used while assuming a coagulation factor concentration of 100%. However, since the optimal administration rate varies greatly among individuals, it is better to monitor the activated partial thromboplastin time (APTT) and the coagulation factor concentration at an early stage. It is also important to check the status of syringe pumps and tubes regularly. Regardless of which method is chosen, when there is a large amount of bleeding, it is necessary not only to supplement the deficient factor but also to replenish other coagulation factors as well as healthy subjects. It is important to understand the advantages and disadvantages of the BI and the CI methods, so as to adopt the method suitable for the individual clinical site and as per the reference guidelines.

4. Important considerations for the use of the continuous administration (CI) method

Even if the target coagulation factor level is set and perioperative management with CI method is executed as planned, the coagulation factor level may not rise as expected. The reason for this may be that the coagulation factor adheres to the surface of the drip tube wall and the assumed dose is not administered. Since the formulations currently used do not include proteins such as albumin, there is a possibility that coagulation factors are lost due to being adsorbed on the tube wall surface when diluted. Therefore, in the case of the CI method, it is necessary to perform injections from the side tube as close to the patient side of the line as possible. During implementation of the CI method, the coagulation factor formulation is placed at room temperature for several hours; this implies that this protein preparation is placed in a harsh environment for an extended period, which makes it difficult to determine the dilution of the preparation and the exact amount that the patient receives. Since the amount of coagulation factor contained in one vial is large, if the preparation is intended to be administered continuously at the determined concentration, the flow rate is usually adjusted to be low, which may result in clogging of the tubes. In order to solve this problem, the use of a low-concentration formulation such as that of 250 or 500 units is advised. We conclude that the CI method can be performed relatively safely by carefully selecting the appropriate formulation.

5. Intraoperative and postoperative management

Measurement of APTT and factor VIII activity is the most common measurement performed during surgery and postoperative procedures. However, in many institutions, there is delay in obtaining the results of the factor VIII activity tests after sample submission, and thus, APTT is considered to be the most useful way to monitor patient condition, especially during surgery. APTT is helpful if there is not much bleeding. However, if the coagulation factor activity other than that of factor VIII decreases, such as when significant bleeding occurs, APTT may not be normalized even if factor VIII is adequately administered. Changes in APTT are thus difficult to interpret, since APTT is affected by the magnitude of the bleeding volume and also by the degree of liver cirrhosis. However, whether the APTT is within the control level can be evaluated, unless it is extremely extended. In cases where it is not possible to obtain hemostasis either intraoperatively or after surgery despite administration of factors VIII and IX, hemophilia may be assumed as the cause, and treatment for this condition may be instituted. If coagulation factor activities other than those of factor VIII and factor IX are low as in splenectomy for cirrhosis of the liver or when the amount of bleeding is large, levels of other coagulation factors may also decrease. Therefore, when and how much fresh frozen plasma (FFP) is administered should be considered separately.

6. Joint surgery

Due to recent advancements in coagulation factor replacement therapy, it is now possible to prevent intra-articular bleeding right from infancy in children with hemophilia. It is thus possible to prevent escalation of hemophilic arthropathy in such children. On the other hand, if hemophilic synovitis has already occurred and several joints show intra-articular bleeding, arthropathy cannot be prevented, and its progress becomes an issue of concern. In joints with advanced arthropathy, degeneration cannot be avoided, even if subsequent bleeding can be completely prevented. Such degeneration of joints is a major cause of physical dysfunction in adult hemophilia patients. Hemophilic arthropathy is commonly seen in the joints of the elbows, knees, and ankles; in particular, dysfunction of lower limb joints greatly affects daily life. Orthopedic treatments for hemophilic arthropathy include measures against intra-articular bleeding, synovitis, and arthropathy. Specific orthopedic treatments are performed for treating synovitis, such as joint puncture, washing, bleeding, synovial membrane resection for the blood remaining in joints, synovial membrane resection and arthrosis, and artificial joint replacement or arthrodesis. Joint puncture and washing are useful treatment methods and are possible outpatient procedures. In the following sections, we discuss synovectomy, artificial joints, and joint fixation in more detail.

7. Synovectomy

Joints that show recurrent intra-articular bleeding on diagnostic images but do not show arthropathy are the best indications for synovial resection. There are two major methods of synovectomy, namely, arthroscopic synovectomy (AS) and open synovectomy. Synovial restoration is a method of restoring the synovial membrane by injecting chemical substances (mainly corticosteroids and antibiotics) and radioactive isotopes into joints. Chemical synoviothesis uses chemical substances and results in severe joint pain after the injection; additionally, it is ineffective despite multiple injections to the joints. However, because it is inexpensive, it is frequently performed in developing countries. Radioactive isotope synovectomy (radioactive synoviothesis) is a treatment that can be expected to be effective with a single intra-articular injection, and it is internationally positioned as the first-line therapy for treatment of hemophilic arthritis. In this therapy modality, only beta rays with a shallow arrival depth are generated, and nuclides with a very short half-life are used. The effect of radioactive synoviothesis on genetic material and the articular cartilage have been reported by several publications, and its safety has been reviewed. However, two cases of leukemia have occurred after synovectomy using P^{32}-labeled radionuclides [2], and in 2010, the Medical and Scientific Advisory Council (MASDAC) issued a cautionary note against the application of radioactive isotopes for synovial treatment [3]. Since arthroscopic synovectomy requires hospitalization and the use of adequate coagulation factor preparations, it is generally applied in cases where at least three cycles of radioactive synoviothesis have been ineffective. However, in Japan, arthroscopic synovectomy is the first choice of treatment. An advantage of this method is that other treatments can be added to the treatment regimen; in addition, this method also allows for the observation of the joint surface. It is recommended that arthroscopic synovectomy be performed even in early arthropathy. Invasive synovectomy is a surgical procedure which involves opening the joint capsule and observing the joint under direct vision, so that a wide expanse of the synovium can be removed in a short time. However, the degree of bleeding also increases, and administration of coagulation factor preparations may be necessary to enable installation of artificial joints. In addition, there is also a high risk of contracture after surgery, and thus, this procedure is not frequently performed.

8. Purpose and significance of synovectomy

Intra-articular bleeding caused by severe hemophilia leads to severe swelling of the joints, and the mobility of the affected limb is limited due to pain. When bleeding events happen repeatedly, the synovial membrane proliferates. Treating hematomas and hemosiderin that occur in joints provides relief, but the blood vessels may re-appear on the synovial membrane; the synovial membrane assumes a villous shape and bleeds easily in such conditions. A vicious circle may be established in which synovial proliferation worsens as bleeding events occur more frequently. The joint, which shows repeated bleeding events, is called a target joint, and the ankle and knee joints in the lower limb and the elbow joint in the upper limb are commonly observed to be target joints. Chronic synovitis eventually causes articular cartilage and subchondral bone erosion and degeneration, resulting in a condition called hemophilic arthropathy. The patient does not use the affected limb either consciously or unconsciously due to pain avoidance, and the functional deterioration progresses with increasing intensity in combination with muscle weakness [4]. Synovial resection is one way to break this vicious circle. As mentioned above, synovial tissue, which shows a villous configuration, bleeds easily; however, if such tissue is surgically removed and appropriate hemostasis is maintained in conjunction with coagulation management, joints can be restored to a state in which they do not easily bleed. However, since synovial excision cannot be recommended until cartilage damage is observed or compatible destroyed joint repair, there are few therapeutic options for highly advanced severe hemophilic arthropathy. Treatment in early-stage hemophilic arthropathy is aimed at providing pain relief by reducing the bleeding frequency; further, this treatment is also applied to delay the progression of arthropathy. However, since the elbow joint does not always receive a high load as compared with the joints of the lower limbs such as the knee joints, if the range of motion can be maintained with little pain or bleeding, synovial ablation is significantly beneficial. Synovial ablation is a good treatment option especially for young people with excellent bone neogenesis and tissue remodeling ability; in this patient population, remodeling may occur on the joint surface depending on the site and stage, and joint repair may also take place to some extent [5, 6].

9. Surgical methods

9.1 Direct surgery

Although different approaches exist for joint surgery, joint synovectomy under direct vision is a common orthopedic surgical procedure and requires no special techniques or instruments. However, post-surgery, synovial membrane remnants may facilitate the recurrence of intra-articular bleeding; surgical removal of the synovial membrane in the joint may also lead to joint contracture caused by postoperative scar formation. In the case of the elbow, if a thorough resection of the synovial membrane in the joint is attempted, the radial head may also have to be removed; both internal and external approaches to the joint may have to be explored. Although there are few opportunities for joint hemorrhage after surgery and hence patient activity increases, there are few things that may improve elbow flexion and extension range. Improvement of forearm restraint can be expected if radial head resection is also performed [7].

9.2 Arthroscopic surgery

Arthroscopy is a surgical procedure that allows surgical access to joints in a minimally invasive fashion and was introduced in the 1940s. Surgical procedures have benefited from advancements in hardware such as cameras, monitors, and surgical instruments. Because there is less damage to the surrounding joint tissues, arthroscopic surgery results in fewer contractures as compared to under-sight surgery. Due to the presence of critically important neural blood vessel bundles surrounding joints, a strong knowledge of anatomy and technical proficiency are required to perform this surgical procedure. However, if done well, synovial resection with arthroscopy can be as effective as or more effective than that performed under direct vision; additionally, as mentioned above, there is little contracture after surgery. Therefore, arthroscopic surgery is recommended for surgical synovectomy of the hemophilic elbow joint [8].

9.2.1 Elbow arthroscopic surgery

The elbow joint has a complicated structure in which the upper and side surfaces of the radius are in contact with the hinge joint (called the arm slider). In order to remove all proliferating synovial membranes in this joint cavity, three parts need to be approached: the anterior, posterior, and the radial parts. It is necessary to create at least two portals for inserting the arthroscope and other instruments such as a shaver. Surgery is performed after the arthroscope and other instruments have been placed properly. Using the abovementioned portal, instruments such as a shaver and a high frequency cautery/transpiration device are employed for performing the surgery. In hemophilic arthropathy, the synovial membrane appears yellowish brown due to hemosiderin deposition caused by repetitive bleeding; the blood vessels in the synovial membrane proliferate significantly in the acute inflammatory phase and bleed easily. However, if the exposed blood vessels are cauterized intraoperatively, the surgery itself is comparable to a conventional synovectomy. It is impossible to surgically remove 100% of the synovial membrane; at the elbow joint, this membrane often grows around both side margins of the wrist joint and around the radial neck. MRI imaging of the synovial membrane is thus performed before surgery, so that a comprehensive resection of the synovium may be achieved to the extent possible. At the end of surgery, one of the portals is used to indwell a closed-type drain in the joint, and the blood in the joint is aspirated and discharged. The drain is removed at about 48–72 hours post-surgery, which is slightly longer than that for conventional arthroscopic surgery.

10. Perioperative hemostasis/coagulation management in synovectomy

Coagulation factor supplementation is frequently performed before surgery, and the aim is strict hemostasis/coagulation management, so that intra-articular bleeding is prevented during the perioperative period. Synovectomy is also specifically aimed at reducing the frequency of intra-articular bleeding. Perioperative bleeding causes synovial proliferation in the joints leading to recurrent bleeding episodes; hence, it is desirable to adequately replenish coagulation factors while monitoring clotting factors and hemostatic and coagulation parameters.

11. Artificial joint replacement

Indications for artificial joint replacement include (1) late-stage arthropathy, (2) serious disruption in activities of daily living (ADL) due to arthropathy, and (3) adults (epiphyseal line is closed). The three points mentioned above are important for patient selection. For the clinical evaluation of late-stage hemophilic arthropathy, the same criteria as applied for osteoarthritis can be accepted. While effect on ADL is an important selection criterion, ADL parameters are highly subjective. Therefore, it is necessary to discuss before surgery whether the patient's desired postoperative life level can be secured. In adult hemophilia patients, it is necessary to explain that when multiple joints develop terminal arthropathy, multiple joint surgeries need to be performed. Artificial joints are usually installed in those aged 60 years or older, and at this age, re-replacement surgery may not be required. However, in some hemophilia cases, patients are forced to use a wheelchair from the age of 20 years, because of pain from arthritis. While artificial joint replacement surgery in young patients does not address the underlying arthritic condition, this surgery nevertheless becomes a necessity to improve QOL. It is important to note that performing re-replacement surgeries repeatedly is not feasible and performing artificial joint replacement may just postpone the occurrence of joint problems. However, in our opinion, living in a wheelchair in the older age may be an acceptable way of maintaining a patient's QOL, if an active lifestyle is facilitated for the patient during the young-to-mature years. For this reason, it may be better to perform artificial joint replacement even in young patients, based on the case details. The most important reason to perform artificial joint replacement is to eliminate or alleviate pain. Simultaneous synovectomy is also performed for cases with joint hemorrhage, so as to stop or reduce the number of bleeding events. On the other hand, the knee joint has been reported to show poor improvement in range of motion. For this reason, postoperative rehabilitation is important.

12. Arthrodesis

Arthrodesis involves surgically immobilizing affected joints. By sacrificing the range of motion of the joint, this procedure treats joint pain and intra-articular bleeding. This procedure is performed primarily on the ankle joint. In the natural course of hemophilic ankylosis, the joints appear stark on diagnostic images in the terminal stage. Therefore, surgery to fix joints artificially is not actively carried out, and numerous parameters are monitored while the patient is administered with symptomatic treatment. Arthrodesis has recently been reviewed as a method for treating artificial ankle joints. Although the treatment protocol varies depending on the facility, if only one side presents with terminal arthrosis, the joint function can be compensated by the other healthy side, so that joint fixation is applied. If ankle joints on both sides are candidates for artificial ankle joint replacement, this condition is an indication for artificial ankle replacement.

13. Problems other than hemostasis in joint surgery

13.1 Preoperative examination and anesthesia management

Spinal anesthesia has been conventionally contraindicated as a method of anesthesia in hemophiliac patients, and surgery has been performed with general anesthesia. The reason is that when the spinal venous plexus is damaged at the needle tip of the lumbar puncture needle, if the coagulation is insufficient, hemorrhage is prolonged and may lead to a deep hematoma; the discovery of such a hematoma is liable to be delayed due to the depth of the location. If such a hematoma occurs, there is a high risk for spinal cord injury. With modern hemostatic management methods, it is possible to maintain the levels of coagulation factors adequately while concurrently administering spinal anesthesia, and if persistent subdural anesthesia can be performed, it is effective for postoperative pain management. However, while very few institutions use spinal anesthesia during surgery in patients with hemophilia, most perform surgery with general anesthesia. There is no relevance of hemophiliac status on the choice of anesthetics. However, depending on the type of antiviral drugs used for people infected with HIV, care should be taken because some drugs inhibit the metabolism of anesthetics and increase the required dosage.

13.2 Surgery in HCV- and HIV-infected patients

Some patients who undergo orthopedic surgery (especially that of artificial knee replacement) show co-occurring HCV or HIV infections due to phytotoxicity. While a proportion of patients with successful treatments (e.g., interferon therapy) no longer have HCV infections, many patients show progression to liver cancer or liver cirrhosis due to long disease duration. In contrast, though symptomatic improvement may be achieved with the latest antiviral drugs in HIV-infected patients, a cure is not possible. Particularly with respect to hepatitis C, postoperative death cases are significantly higher among cases characterized as Child classification B, those with low ascites and albumin, and those with thrombocytopenia [9]. Confirmation of these conditions is important for surgical decisions.

13.3 Prevention of deep venous thrombosis (DVT)

Lower extremity artificial joint surgery is one of the risk factors for deep venous thrombosis (DVT), and DVT risk is of particular relevance in hemophilia patients. However, most hemophilia patients undergoing artificial joint replacement surgery are adolescents on anti-inflammatory analgesic therapy and show no other comorbidities that may influence thrombus development. Therefore, the risk of DVT occurrence due to lower extremity artificial joint surgery may be lower than that due to general lower limb prosthesis replacement surgery. However, it was reported that among asymptomatic patients, DVT was detected by lower limb ultrasonography in 10% of cases after surgery, even in patients with hemophilia [10]. A previous report has suggested that in addition to physical methods such as application of elastic stockings and intermittent pneumatic compression, anticoagulation therapy is administered at about half of the facilities where the survey was conducted [11]. Either way, even in patients with hemophilia, physicians must be alert to the development of postoperative DVT, and timely cessation of prescribed bed rest and early rehabilitation are important.

14. Latest findings due to the appearance of half-life extended drugs

The development of coagulation factor preparations is one of the most important factors impacting the prognosis and quality of life of patients with hemophilia. Recent advancements in extending the half-life of drugs using various mechanisms have attracted much attention. Such extended half-life formulations make it possible to reduce the frequency of self-injections even in regular prophylaxis therapy and reduce the frequency of bleeding symptoms (such as bleeding in the joints and muscles). In addition, such advancements not only extend the half-life and improve the stability of the drugs; they also impact patient burden by reducing the number of required hospital visits. Various benefits have been obtained from the use of half-life extended drugs, and this development has brought about major changes in the treatment of hemophilia. However, since half-life extended medicines are short, there is a lack of substantial evidence of the efficacy in perioperative administration regimens. Moreover, the number of cases in which these drugs have been used is too small for inclusion in case report studies. In this regard, we have experienced and reported a case of perioperative management of hemophilia A using efraloctocog alfa (ELOCTATE®) during endoscopic nasal pituitary adenomectomy for growth hormone-producing pituitary adenoma. There are no other reports of the successful use of ELOCTATE (a drug with an extended half-life) in conjunction with the BI method for a major surgery. We summarize below details of the case study [12]. A 28-year-old man was admitted to our hospital due to bulging of the glabella. He had first noticed the bulging of the glabella in 2013. He was aware of the enlargement of his fingers and the size of his shoes since August 2016, and he was now seeking medical attention. He was referred to the department of endocrinology and metabolism at our hospital with suspected acromegaly. A diagnosis of growth hormone-producing pituitary adenoma was made by performing several tests, including a brain MRI and loading tests. Furthermore, we decided to perform endoscopic nasal pituitary adenomectomy at our department of neurosurgery. The patient clinical history included hemophilia A, pediatric asthma, and hypothyroidism.

Hemophilia A was diagnosed as moderate in infancy. The patient reported self-injecting rurioctocog alfa (trade name: ADVATE®) two to three times a week for hemophilia. The final bleeding episode occurred in the left knee joint in April 2013 and required hospitalization for 3 days. Factor VIII inhibitors were not detectable in the patient's blood. We prepared a regimen for administration of rFVIIIFc in accordance with guidelines for hemostasis treatment for hemophilia patients without inhibitors (Revision 2013, published by the Japanese society of Thrombosis and Hemostasis). At our hospital, the results of factor VIII activity cannot be obtained promptly, so in the perioperative period, we monitored APTT in lieu of factor VIII levels in sera. From day 2 onward, we injected rFVIIIFc intravenously at 2 PM daily and measured APTT and factor VIII activity at 6 AM the following morning (16 hours after intravenous injection). A blood test was conducted to measure APTT and factor VIII activity at 6 AM on surgery day. On the day of the surgery, 4000 IU of rFVIIIFc were intravenously injected at 8 AM (1 hour before leaving the ward for the surgery), and APTT and factor VIII activity were measured again after 15 minutes of intravenous injection (because peak levels of rFVIIIFc in the blood are achieved approximately 15 minutes after intravenous injection). APTT at this time was assumed to be a function primarily of factor VIII activity and was used as the most important index in perioperative control. The surgery began at 10:14 AM and ended at 1:39 PM (3 hours and 25 minutes). The surgery performed was an endoscopic nasal pituitary adenomectomy. The volume of bleeding during the surgery was 150 ml and was in close agreement with the expected volume of bleeding. Prior to surgery, a risk of bleeding from the nasal mucosa was suspected; however, only two mild nasal bleeding events were confirmed and were resolved adequately. The patient was discharged on day 13, on schedule. Thus, perioperative management using drugs with an extended half-life can be applied to control hemostasis/coagulation at the perioperative stage using the BI method even for major surgery, as in the case described above. The advantage of perioperative management by the BI method using half-life extended drugs is that these drugs need to be administered through intravenous injection only once a day, and such a treatment protocol is easy to perform at a hospital. Furthermore, the BI method is also economical as it reduces the amount and thus the cost of the drug, as compared with the CI method using the existing coagulation factor preparations. For perioperative management using extended half-life drugs, we consider that further case studies are necessary to prepare dosing regimens. However, such drugs have the potential to impact not only periodic replacement therapy but also perioperative management in hemophilia patients. For the reasons stated above, we feel that the extended half-life drugs have the potential to significantly impact hemophilia treatment.

15. Possibility of subcutaneously injectable coagulation factor preparations

Another recent advancement in hemophilia drugs is the development of a subcutaneously injectable formulation, which overcomes the need for intravenous injection. The common name of this drug is emicizumab, and the trade name is HEMLIBRA®. The efficacy of emicizumab is characterized as "suppression of bleeding tendency in congenital factor VIII-deficient patients positive for inhibitors against factor VIII." As with other factor VIII drugs and bypass medicines, there are no indications for administration during perioperative period or during sudden bleeding events, and increase in blood emicizumab levels is disallowed. Currently, this drug has been formulated as an intravenous injection and is being used for sudden bleeding events or during surgery in patients who undergo prophylactic replacement therapy with subcutaneous coagulation factor preparations. In the future, it is expected that this drug will also be recommended for use in hemophilia patients who are negative for factor VIII inhibitors. However, currently, this drug is being administered only to patients positive for factor VIII inhibitors. Phase III clinical trials of the use of emicizumab in surgical cases have been conducted, but the subjects have been limited to those positive for factor VIII inhibitors. Literature evidence of the use of emicizumab during surgery in patients without inhibitors is lacking, and thus comparative assessments cannot be made. There is also no evidence regarding the use of this drug during time of surgery in patients with inhibitors as well. As described above, there is little evidence to support the efficacy of emicizumab administration in perioperative period, and further studies are indicated.

16. Treatment of hemophiliac patients with inhibitors

16.1 Outline

Inhibitors are anti-factor VIII or anti-factor IX allogeneic antibodies generated against factor VIII and factor IX in pharmaceutical preparations as a result of replacement therapy with coagulation factor preparations. When an inhibitor generates, it binds to factor VIII and factor IX, resulting in structural and functional abnormalities. Furthermore, as the clearance is increased by the formation of the antigen-antibody complex, the hemostatic effect of replacement therapy drastically decreases/disappears [13]. Hemostasis therapy is roughly divided into neutralization therapy and bypass hemostasis therapy. And it is chosen mainly based on the severity of bleeding symptoms, the potency and reactivity of the inhibitor, and past medical history.

16.2 Inhibitor phenotype

Inhibitors are measured by Bethesda method [14] based on coagulation single step method. The amount of antibody that inactivates factor VIII or factor IX contained in 1 ml of normal plasma by 50% is defined as 1 Bethesda Unit/ml (BU/ml). Normally, >0.6 BU/ml is judged to be positive for inhibitors. In particular, the Nijmegen method is recommended for measurements around 1 BU/ml [15]. Inhibitor titers are defined as high titer ≧ 5 BU/ml and low titer <5 BU/ml. A high responder (HR) is defined as a case in which an inhibitor of ≧5 BU/ml in the Factor VIII/IX Subcommittee of the International Conference on Thrombosis and Hemostasis. And it is recommended that <5 BU/ml case be defined as low responder (LR) [16]. Inhibitor titers may jump sharply 5–7 days after preparation administration. This is called an anamnestic response. The Japan Society of Thrombosis and Hemostasis Academic Standardization Committee Hemophilia Subcommittee advocates an algorithm for selecting therapeutic preparations depending on the potency of the inhibitor and either HR or LR.

17. Replacement therapy

17.1 Selection criteria for replacement therapy and dosage

The first choice of low titer (<5 BU/ml) inhibitor holding LR with no anamnestic response in the past is a continuation of replacement therapy [17]. To obtain a definite hemostatic effect, add the necessary formulation for inhibitor neutralization and target hemostatic level. The neutralization amount (unit) is theoretically calculated as 40 × weight (kg) × {[100 hematocrit value (%)]/100} × inhibitor titer (BU/ml). Depending on the inactivation pattern of the anti-factor VIII or anti-IX factor activity of the inhibitor, it may not necessarily rise as expected. Therefore, monitoring of coagulation factor activity is desired. Bypass hemostasis therapy described later is the first choice for HR types that have elevated ≧ 5 BU/ml in the past even at <5 BU/ml, but in case of severe bleeding symptoms or major surgery, replacement therapy is selected. However, in the case of HR, it is practical to plan a hemostasis therapy after the reaction, taking into consideration the appearance of previous immune response after 5–7 days after administration. Usually change to bypass hemostasis therapy. Even when the inhibitor titer is 5–10 BU/ml, it is possible to carry out neutralization therapy with high volumes of Factor VIII and Factor IX preparation at severe bleeding and major surgery.

17.2 Selection of replacement therapy preparation

There are three types of factor VIII (FVIII) preparations that can be used in Japan. They are plasma-derived factor VIII formulation, genetically modified factor VIII, and plasma-derived factor VIII (FVIII)/von Willebrand factor (VWF) complex preparation. There are two types of factor IX preparation that can be used: plasma-derived preparations and recombinant preparations. In some hemophilia A inhibitor cases, it is known that the hemostatic effect of the FIII/VWF preparation exceeds that of the factor VIII preparation. It is clarified that this inhibitor is an antibody which recognizes the factor VIII light chain and suppresses FVIII/VWF binding, and reactivity to FVIII is decreased by the presence of VWF [18].

17.3 Method of administration of preparation

Normally, factor VIII preparation and factor IX preparation are administered in bolus, but continuous administration is also selected at severe bleeding and hemostatic management of major operation. There are no standards for dose administration in inhibitor cases. If the inhibitor is completely neutralized by the initial bolus administration, the coagulation factor activity can theoretically be maintained in the administration example similar to the cases without inhibitor. In practice, however, higher doses are often required.

18. Bypass hemostatic therapy

According to the guidelines published by the Japan Thrombosis Hemorrhagic Society, the first choice when the inhibitor titer ≧ 5 BU/ml is bypass hemostasis therapy except severe bleeding symptoms and hemostasis management during major surgery [17]. Traditionally, activated prothrombin complex concentrates (aPCC) or prothrombin complex concentrates (PCC) were the main body of bypass hemostasis therapy, but bypass hemostasis therapy has greatly advanced after the introduction of genetically modified active factor VII factor formulation (rFVIIa). Sales of PCC preparations adapted for inhibitors have been discontinued. Currently available bypass preparations are three, aPCC (FEIBA®), rFVIIa (NovoSeven®), and blood coagulation factor X factor-activated factor VII (Byclot®).

18.1 Bypass hemostatic therapy preparation

18.1.1 Activated prothrombin complex concentrates (aPCC)

18.1.1.1 Hemostasis management during surgery by aPCC

Conventionally, it was extremely difficult for a variety of reasons to perform hemostasis management at the time of surgery of HR inhibitor cases with inhibitors of high titer by only aPCC. The main reasons are the uncertainty of the hemostatic effect, expensive medical expenses, thrombosis, and fear of onset of disseminated intravascular coagulation syndrome (DIC), and furthermore, the evidence is low. Many of the cases used aPCC in combination after neutralization therapy with factor VIII and factor IX preparations. However, in conjunction with the increase in patients undergoing surgery by rFVIIa, reports on practical cases with only aPCC have been increasing in recent years. According to a multicenter retrospective study by Negrier et al., aPCC was used for 19 small surgical procedures [19]. The most frequent cases were joint puncture (10 cases), the number of doses was two to six times, and the administration days were in the range of 2–4 days, both of which were effective. The dose was 78–160 units/kg/day. Four cases were used for tooth extraction, three cases were administered twice, one case was administered six times, and the administration period was, respectively, 1 day and 3 days. Four cases were performed in major surgery. The breakdown was knee joint synovectomy, knee arthroplasty, skin muscle formation, and prostatectomy. The dose and duration of aPCC during major surgery differ depending on the operation name. The dose is 120–210 units/kg/day and the administration period is 5–21 days. The dosing regimen after surgical treatment such as subcutaneously implanted central intravenous catheterization procedure ranged from 50 to 74 units/kg one to two times/day; dosing days ranged from 1 to 6 days [20]. In Japan, since aPCC had limitation of use (inhibitor potency ≥10 BU/ml, within 3 days of administration), experience of using aPCC in major surgery is small. Since these restrictions have been removed since 2008, surgical therapy using aPCC in Japan could be considered. The number of cases is still small internationally, and it is necessary to standardize on the aPCC administration regimen at the time of surgery in the future.

18.1.1.2 Anamnestic response by aPCC

A fragment of factor VIII is detected in aPCC. Therefore, there are cases in which inhibitor titers are increased by repeated administration of aPCC. This is because aPCC contains the light chain fragment of factor VIII, and it is common in inhibitors of the light chain recognition type in particular [21]. Therefore, in cases that the inhibitor titer does not decrease and the high value is sustained, it is necessary to pay attention to the anamnestic response caused by aPCC. Incidentally, even in cases with this history of reaction, there are cases in which they subsequently decline as a result. In the report of Negrier et al., anamnestic response was seen in 31.5% of the patients, but of which 64.7% had gradually decreased [19].

18.1.2 rFVIIa

18.1.2.1 Hemostasis management during surgery by rFVIIa

rFVIIa is being used not only for small surgical operations but also for moderate or more surgical operations. Lusher et al. collected results on 103 surgical operations totaling 21 cases of major operation, 57 cases of small operation, and 25 cases of suturing relation [22]. According to the report, effective cases were 81, 86 and 92%, respectively, indicating that major surgery is also possible with hemostasis management by rFVIIa. Even in Japan, there are no restrictions on insurance medical treatment, so we have used more experience than aPCC and the number of cases such as large orthopedic surgery including artificial joint replacement surgery is increasing. Schrarer et al. recommended that 90 μg/kg every 2–3 days for 1–2 days, in large surgery, and, in small surgery, the same amount of administration every 2–4 hours, every 6–7 days and every 6–8 hours 2 weeks [23]. Rodriguez et al. collected 108 cases of orthopedic surgical cases with inhibitor and reported the usefulness of rFVIIa [24]. Eighty cases of orthopedic surgical cases were collected over the period from 2000 to 2006. The initial dose was 120 μg/kg and thereafter administration of 90 μg/kg every 2 hours or 50 μg/kg/hour in continuous administration. Obergfell et al. reported that this regimen is useful [25]. In Japan's guidelines, as in the case of severe bleeding hemostasis therapy, administration is performed every 2 hours for 1–2 days at the time of major operation. Thereafter, they recommend a regimen that gradually extends the dosing interval, for example, every 3, 4, 8, and 12 hours [17]. Because of its short half-life and the fact that thrombin burst is caused by high concentration of FVIIa is considered to be the basis of hemostatic effect, bolus administration is recommended in principle for administration of rFVIIa. However, there are increasing reports that sustained administration therapy is useful, especially when frequent administration is required as in surgical operation [26, 27]. In general administration method, continuous administration is started at 14–16.5 μg/kg/hour after the initial bolus administration of 90–120 μg/kg. Thereafter, the factor VII activity (FVII:C) is administered so as to maintain at least 10 units/ml. However, Ludlam et al. recently encouraged maintaining the trough level of FVII:C at 30 units/ml at a dose of 50 μg/kg/h during major surgery [28].

18.1.3 Mixture of plasma-derived factor VIIa and factor X (MC710)

MC710 is a plasma-derived new bypass hemostatic therapeutic agent developed in Japan, because the effect of FVIIa is enhanced and sustained due to the coexistence of FX (FVIIa:FX = 1:10). According to pharmacodynamic analysis by coagulation waveform analysis conducted in Phase I study, activated partial thromboplastin time (APTT), maximum solidification rate, and maximum coagulation acceleration peaked 10 minutes after MC 710 administration. And it was before administration level 12 hours after administration. Although the enhancing effect of MC710 was not concentration dependent, it was higher than 120 μg/kg of rFVIIa or 50/75 U/kg of aPCC at dose>80 μg/kg [29]. Furthermore, in Phase II clinical trials, efficacy and safety were examined at two doses of 60 μg/kg and 120 μg/kg in patients with inhibitors of six cases. The hemostasis effect was effective and remarkable 8 hours after administration in total nine bleeding episodes. There were no side effects attributable to the formulation [30].

19. Selection of bypass hemostatic therapy preparation

Both current bypass treatment formulations, aPCC and rFVIIa, have been clarified for efficacy in hemostatic therapy for acute bleeding and surgical treatment. However, as to selection of both formulations, it is necessary to comprehensively select the presence/absence of anamnestic response in the past, the risk of thrombosis, and past hemostatic effect. It was revealed that the hemostasis effect between a single dose of aPCC (75–100 Units/kg) and two doses of rFVIIa (90–120 μg/kg) is equivalent to the hemorrhage of the joint [31]. Interestingly, however, cases were found in which there was a difference in hemostatic effect among the preparations. Even in the same case, the difference in the hemostatic effect between both preparations suggests that it is necessary to change to multiple drugs when the first choice preparation is ineffective [32]. For the selection of preparations at the time of surgery, it has been reported that preparations are added ex vivo to the patient's plasma prior to surgery and the hemostatic effect is judged by rotation thromboelastometry (ROTEM) before operation [33].

20. Bypass hemostatic therapy in special case

20.1 Cases before immune tolerance induction (ITI therapy)

Regarding the effectiveness of ITI therapy, the only statistically proven factor is the potency of the inhibitor at the beginning of ITI. Therefore, the lower the inhibitor titer, the higher the success rate. Recent international clinical studies of ITI also target <10 BU/ml patients [34]. As a rule, rFVIIa is the first choice in cases where anamnestic response occurs with aPCC administration.

20.2 Cases with a history of allergic symptoms

Some patients with hemophilia B with some inhibitors have allergic symptoms for the preparation containing factor IX. Allergic symptoms are often severe and may present anaphylaxis. The essence of allergic symptoms is anti-IX factor IgG (immunoglobulin G), which is said to be particularly IgG1 antibody [35]. The aPCC preparation contains factor IX. Patients who are allergic to factor IX preparation may have similar symptoms to aPCC. For such cases, it is also possible to desensitize by administering a preparation containing factor IX in small amounts [36]. In general, however, the first choice in cases with allergic history is rFVIIa and MC710.

21. Conclusion

Here we summarize the various options available for the perioperative management of patients with hemophilia and also discuss joint surgery, which is an important aspect of treatment of patients with hemophilia. Unlike healthy subjects, patients with hemophilia require special perioperative management. We hope that this manuscript will help in formulating better treatment of patients with hemophilia in the future.

Acknowledgements

We would like to thank Mr. Satoshi Shinmura (pharmacist at Bioverativ Japan) and Mr. Yoichi Hirose (medical representative at Chugai Pharmaceutical Co., Ltd.) who helped with the collection of the thesis and advised on the latest developments in the field.

Conflict of interest

We do not have conflicts of interest to disclose.

Notes/thanks/other declarations

I would like to thank the coauthors who supported the writing of this chapter and advised me.

Author details

Atsushi Okamoto, Kenta Yamamoto, Go Eguchi, Yoshitaka Kanai, Terufumi Yamaguchi and Yasuhiro Maeda*
Department of Hematology, National Hospital Organization Osaka Minami Medical Center, Osaka, Japan

*Address all correspondence to: ymaeda@ommc-hp.jp

IntechOpen

© 2018 The Author(s). Licensee IntechOpen. This chapter is distributed under the terms of the Creative Commons Attribution License (http://creativecommons.org/licenses/by/3.0), which permits unrestricted use, distribution, and reproduction in any medium, provided the original work is properly cited.

References

[1] Amano K. Hemostasis Management of the Latest Haemophilia. Tokyo: Medical Plactice 24 Bunkodo; 2007. pp. 2165-2170

[2] Dunn AL, Manco-Johnson M, Busch MT, et al. Leukemia and P32 radionuclide synovectomy for hemophilic arthropathy. Journal of Thrombosis and Haemostasis. 2005;**3**:1541-1542

[3] Medical and Scientific Advisory Council: MASAC Recommendation #194. 2010. Available from: http://www.hemophilia.org/NHFWeb/MainPgs/MainNHF.aspx?menuid=156&contentid=335

[4] Taketani H. Orthopedic treatment for haemophilic arthropathy. Blood Frontier. 2006;**16**:1797-1804

[5] Tanaka Y, Shinohara Y, Narikawa K, et al. Arthroscopic synovectomies combined with reduced weight-bearing using patella tendonbearing braces were very effective for progressed haemophilic ankle arthropathy in three paediatric patients. Haemophilia. 2009;**15**:833-836

[6] Shimada K, Takedani H, Inoue K, et al. Arthroscopic synovectomy of the elbow covered with rFVIIa in a Haemophilia B juvenile with inhibitor. Haemophilia. 2012;**18**:e414-e416

[7] Lofqvist T, Nilsson IM, Petersson C. Orthopaedic surgery in hemophilia. Clinical Orthopaedics and Related Research. 1996;**332**:232-241

[8] Journeycake JM, Miller KL, Anderson AM, et al. Arthroscopic synovectomy in children and adolescents with hemophilia. Journal of Pediatric Hematology/Oncology. 2003;**25**:726-731

[9] Hirose J, Takedani H, Koibuchi T. The risk of elective orthopaedic surgery for haemophilia patients:Japanese single-Centre experience. Haemophilia. 2013;**19**:951-955

[10] Hermans C, Hammer F, Lobet S, et al. Subclinical deep venous thrombosis observed in 10% of hemophilic patients undergoing major orthopedic surgery. Journal of Thrombosis and Haemostasis. 2010;**8**:1138-1140

[11] Hermans C. Venous thromboembolic disease in patients with haemophilia. Thrombosis Research. 2012;**130**(Suppl 1):S50-S52

[12] Okamoto A, Yamamoto K, Eguchi G, et al. Perioperative management of haemophilia A using recombinant factor VIII Fc fusion protein in a patient undergoing endoscopic nasal pituitary adenomectomy for a growth hormone-producing pituitary adenoma. Haemophilia. 2017;**6**:e525-e527. DOI: 10.1111/hae.13347

[13] Shima M. Characterization of factor VIII inhibitors. International Journal of Hematology. 2006;**83**:109-118

[14] Kasper CK, Aledort L, Aronson D, et al. Proceedings: A more uniform measurement of factor VIII inhibitors. Thrombosis et Diathesis Haemorrhagica. 1975;**34**:612

[15] Verbruggen B, Novakova I, Wessels H, et al. The Nijmegen modification of the Bethesda assay for factor VIII; C inhibitors: Improved specificity and reliability. Thrombosis and Haemostasis. 1995;**73**:247-251

[16] White GC 2nd, Rosendaal F, Aledort LM, et al. Definitions in hemophilia. Recommendation of the scientific subcommittee on factor VIII and factor IX of the scientific and standardization committee of the international society on thrombosis and haemostasis. Thrombosis and Haemostasis. 2001;**85**:560

[17] Sakai M, Taki M, Ieko M, et al. Guidelines for hemostasis treatment for congenital hemophilia patients with inhibitors 2013 revised edition. Japanese Journal of Thrombosis and Hemostasis. 2013;**19**:520-539

[18] Inoue T, Shima M, Takeyama M, et al. Higher recovery of factor VIII(FVIII) with intermediate FVIII/von Willebrand factor concentrate than with recombinant FVIII in a haemophilia A patient with an inhibitor. Haemophilia. 2006;**12**:110-113

[19] Negrier C, Goudemand J, Sultan Y, et al. Multicenter retrospective study on the utilization of FEIBA in France in patients with factor VIII and factor IX inhibitors. French FEIBA Study Group. Factor eight bypassing activity. Thrombosis and Haemostasis. 1997;**77**:1113-1119

[20] Kraut EH, Aledort LM, Arkin S, et al. Surgical interventions in a cohort of patients with haemophilia A and inhibitors: An experiential retrospective chart review. Haemophilia. 2007;**13**:508-517

[21] Yoshioka A, Kamisue S, Tanaka I, et al. Anamnestic response following infusion of prothrombin complex concentrates (PCC) and activated prothrombin complex concentrates (aPCC) in hamophilia A patients with inhibitors. Blood Coagulation and Fibrinolysis. 1991;**2**:51-58

[22] Lusher JM, Roberts HR, Davignon G, et al. A randomized, double-blind comparison of two dosage levels of recombinant factor VIIa in the treatment of joint, muscle and mucocutaneous haemorrhages in persons with haemophilia A and B, with and without inhibitors. rFVIIa Study Group. Haemophilia. 1998;**4**:790-798

[23] Scharrer I. Recombinant factor VIIa for patients with inhibitors to factor VIII or IX or factor VIII deficiency. Haemophilia. 1999;**5**:253-259

[24] Rodrigues-Merchan EC, Jd WJ, Wallny T, et al. Elective orthopedic surgery for hemophilia patients with inhibitors: New opportunities. Seminars in Hematology. 2004;**41**(1 Suppl):109-116

[25] Obergfell A, Auvinen MK, Mathew P. Recombinant activated factor VII for haemophilia patients with inhibitors undergoing orthopedic surgery: A review of the literature. Haemophilia. 2008;**14**:233-241

[26] Schulman S, Bech Jensen M, Varon D, et al. Feasibility of using recombinant factor VIIa in continuous infusion. Thrombosis and Haemostasis. 1996;**75**:32-36

[27] Mauser-Bunschoten EP, Koopman MM, Goede-Bolder AD, et al. Efficacy of recombinant factor VIIa administered by continuous infusion to haemophilia patients with inhibitors. Haemophilia. 2002;**8**:649-656

[28] Ludlam CA, Smith MP, Morfini M, et al. A prospective study of recombinant activated factor VII administered by continuous infusion to inhibitor patients undergoing elective major orthopaedic surgery: A pharmacokinetic and efficacy evaluation. British Journal of Haematology. 2003;**120**:808-813

[29] Shirahata A, Fukutake K, Mimaya J, et al. Results of clot waveform analysis and thrombin generation test for a plasma-derived factor VIIa and X mixture (MC710) in haemophilia patients with inhibitors—Phase I trial; 2nd report. Haemophilia. 2013;**19**:330-337

[30] Shirahata A, Fukutake K, Takamatsu J, et al. A phase II clinical trial of a mixture of plasma-derived factor VIIa and factor X (MC710) in haemophilia patients with inhibitors: Haemostatic efficacy, safety and pharmacokinetics/pharmacodynamics. Haemophilia. 2013;**19**:853-860

[31] Astermark J, Donfield SM, DiMichele DM, et al. A randomized comparison of bypassing agents in hemophilia complicated by an inhibitor: The FEIBA NovoSeven Comparative (FENOC) study. Blood. 2007;**109**:546-551

[32] Hayashi T, Tanaka I, Shima M, et al. Unresponsiveness to factor VIII inhibitor bypassing agents during Haemostatic treatment for life-threatening massive bleeding in a patient with haemophilia A and a high responding inhibitor. Haemophilia. 2004;**10**:397-400

[33] Furukawa S, Nogami K, Ogiwara K, et al. Systematic monitoring of hemostatic management in hemophilia A patients with inhibitor in the perioperative period using rotational thromboelastometry. Journal of Thrombosis and Haemostasis. 2015;**13**:1279-1284

[34] Hay CR, Dimichele DM. International immnne tolerance study: The principal results of the international immune tolerance study: A randomized dose comparison. Blood. 2012;**119**:1335-1344

[35] Sawamoto Y, Shima M, Yamamoto M, et al. Measurement of anti-factor IX IgG subclasses in haemophilia B patients who developed inhibitors with episodes of allergic reactions to factor IX concentrates. Thrombosis Research. 1996;**83**:279-286

[36] Shibata M, Shima M, Misu H, et al. Management of haemophilia B inhibitor patients with anaphylactic reactions to FIX concentrates. Haemophilia. 2003;**9**:269-271

Chapter 4

Clinical Issues in Women with Inherited Bleeding Disorders

Ana-Rebeca Jaloma-Cruz, Isaura-Araceli González-Ramos, Diana Ornelas-Ricardo, Clara-Ibet Juárez-Vázquez and Hilda Luna-Záizar

Abstract

Various inherited bleeding disorders deserve careful medical management due to their implications in women's health. In both hemophilia A and B, almost exclusively, males are affected while carrier females are generally asymptomatic. Nevertheless, carriers may present important bleeding tendencies, which can eventually constitute a serious threat to life, especially after surgery or postpartum. In addition, in rare but significant cases, some genetic mechanisms have been found to cause hemophilia in females. Aside from von Willebrand disease, which is the most widespread and better described hemorrhagic condition in women, platelet disorders and some rare clotting deficiencies cause a wide variety of mucocutaneous bleedings, menorrhagia, or postpartum bleeding, hence constituting an important health risk. A review of the genetic and pathophysiological aspects as well as main clinical complications of all these conditions will allow for preventive practices aimed at improving the quality of life of women with bleeding disorders.

Keywords: symptomatic carriers and women with hemophilia, von Willebrand disease, platelet disorders, rare bleeding disorders, bleedings in pregnancy and postpartum

1. Introduction

Inherited bleeding disorders are a group of deficiencies including the decreased function or number of platelets (thrombocytopenia) and clotting factor deficiencies, mainly von Willebrand disease (VWD), hemophilia A (HA), and hemophilia B (HB), as well as rare bleeding disorders (RBDs) such as deficiencies of factors (F) I (fibrinogen), II, FV, combined FV-FVIII, FVII, FX, FXI, and FXIII and congenital deficiency of vitamin K-dependent factors and plasminogen activator inhibitor (PAI-1). Mostly autosomal recessive, together they have a prevalence of 1:500,000 to 1:1–3 million in the general population [1, 2].

Although all these entities cause bleeding tendencies in the affected males or females, there are relevant clinical issues related to obstetric and gynecological conditions that require special considerations in their management [1].

Menorrhagia or the more precise term of heavy menstrual bleeding (HMB) recommended by the International Federation of Gynecology and Obstetrics (FIGO)

IntechOpen

is the most common symptom in women with bleeding disorders and is defined as bleeding that lasts more than 7 days or results in the loss of more than 80 mL of blood per menstrual cycle [1, 3]. In terms of women's quality of life, HMB is defined as "the excessive menstrual blood loss which interferes with the woman's physical, emotional, social and material quality of life, and can occur alone or in combination with other symptoms; HMB is typically associated with a symptom complex, including variable pelvic pain and somatic symptoms" [3].

The FIGO also classifies the dysfunctional uterine bleeding disorders and identifies impaired hemostasis as one of the three recognized causes [3]. More than 70% of women with VWD present HMB and they are five times more likely to suffer from this complication than women without the condition. As for platelet disorders, the prevalence of HMB is 51% in women with Bernard-Soulier syndrome and 98% in women with Glanzmann thrombasthenia. HMB is present in 59% of women with FXI deficiency, in 57% of hemophilia carriers, and in 35–70% of women with other rare factor deficiencies [1].

In addition to HMB, women with bleeding disorders frequently suffer from large clots and flooding during their menstruation as well as bleeds after their menstrual period, conditions that may seriously affect their quality of life. Since 1990, Higham et al. proposed a pictorial blood assessment chart (PBAC) that was based on a validation study against the alkaline hematin method for blood measurement, which is known to be very accurate and reproducible but not practical in routine clinical use [4]. A score greater than 100, based on the number of used tampons or towels and the points assigned according to the estimated blood soaking, represents a very good prediction and considers a menstrual blood loss of more than 80 mL as positive HMB. The passage of clots and flooding episodes are also registered and considered for the score [1, 4].

HMB can be considered a significant symptom of a bleeding disorder, especially when it is present at menarche. The hematological evaluation of women with HMB should take into account the personal and familial bleeding history of epistaxis, easy bruising bleeding in the oral cavity, prolonged bleeding following dental extraction, unexpected post-surgical bleeding, hemorrhage requiring transfusion, and postpartum hemorrhage, especially after 24 h [1]. In patients with at least 2–3 symptoms, additional screening and confirmatory tests for VWD, platelet function, coagulation times, and clotting factor levels are mandatory [1].

Concerning the management of pregnancy and postpartum, women suspected of having a bleeding disorder or being a carrier of hemophilia should undergo diagnostic testing before getting pregnant in order to receive appropriate preconception counseling and early pregnancy management. This information allows for consideration of the available reproductive choices and options for prenatal diagnosis such as planning for pregnancy and establishing the best management in terms of hemostatic treatment and for the support of the pregnancy [1]. After the delivery, the elevated coagulation factor returns to the pre-pregnancy levels; therefore, the main risk of bleeding is after miscarriage or delivery. Postpartum hemorrhage (PPH) is a major cause of maternal morbidity and mortality, especially in developing countries or rural regions. PPH accounts for an estimated 140,000 maternal deaths each year worldwide and many women suffer from long-term debilitating consequences of the resultant anemia. Even if the most common causes of PPH are uterine atony, retained placenta, or genital tract trauma, coagulation disorders are also recognized causes of such complication [1].

In the next sections, we summarize clinical generalities, genetic aspects, impact on women's health, recommended treatment, and medical management of common inherited bleeding disorders.

2. Symptomatic hemophilia carriers

2.1 Generalities

Hemophilia is an X-linked disease due to mutations in the genes *F8* and *F9* (causing HA and HB, respectively) and subsequent deficiency of the clotting factors VIII (FVIII) and IX (FIX). HA affects 1/5000–10,000 males and HB 1/30,000 males. Both factors act in the same step of the coagulation mechanism and, when any of them is deficient, a diminished thrombin generation ensues. The symptoms have an inverse correlation with the plasmatic activity of the deficient factor, and the diagnosis and severity classification are based on the residual factor level [5].

2.2 Genetic aspects

Due to its recessive X-linked inheritance, males are mostly affected while the heterozygous female carriers are usually asymptomatic. Although some carriers have various bleeding manifestations and can even express severe (FVIII/FIX <0.01 U mL^{-1}) or moderate (FVIII/FIX 0.01–0.05 U mL^{-1}) phenotypes, their specific clinical manifestations and genetic data have hardly been described [6].

Hemophilia female carriers may be affected by hemorrhagic manifestations due to different genetic conditions: both mutated alleles with homozygous or compound heterozygous mutations in *F8* or *F9* genes, hemizygosity in 45,X (Turner syndrome) patients with a mutated X chromosome, or extremely skewed X-chromosome inactivation pattern (X-IP) in carriers who have inactivated the wild-type allele and thereby have a highly decreased amount of the concerned factor and express the symptoms of the disease [7]. The molecular genetic analysis is essential in elucidating the mechanisms underlying the bleeding phenotype in females with hemophilia [8–10].

In accordance with international estimations, there are 3–5 potential female carriers for each male with hemophilia, but not every carrier knows her genetic status. According to the study of Bernard, only 38% of the potential carriers have been screened about their carrier/non-carrier status. He analyzed 408 potential carriers and reported that only a limited fraction of them received information from a hemophilia specialist about their status and underwent coagulation factor analysis; the remaining large fraction failed to accomplish the screening due to lack of communication within the family and unawareness of the inheritance mode [11].

If women do not realize the possibility of being carriers, all their symptoms can be overlapped with normal women and those with VWD or qualitative platelet disorders [7]; so, all possible or potential carriers must be screened and should be advised about care and surveillance regarding bleeding tendencies [12].

2.3 Clinical features

Different studies have shown the increased tendency of bleeding in hemophilia carriers compared to healthy females. Olsson et al. described the bleeding symptoms in 126 hemophilia carriers in contrast to 90 non-hemophilia carriers; the hemorrhagic tendency was normal in 82 carriers (65%) and in all but two women in the control group (98%). They reported that there was no difference in bleeding symptoms between carriers from hemophiliac families and carriers with sporadic mutations. The proportion of carriers and controls reporting bleeding symptoms was different with statistically significant results ($p < 0.001$), **Table 1** [13].

Paroskie compared 44 HA carriers with 43 healthy women and found a significant ($p < 0.05$) increase in clinical features as shown in **Table 2** [5]. Contrary to

Clinical features	Carriers (%)	Controls (%)
Menorrhagia	37	16
Bleeding from minor wounds	32	0
Surgery	32	7.2
Tooth extraction	30	0
Nosebleed	24	4.4
Cutaneous bleeding	17	1.1

Taken from information reported by Olsson et al. [13].

Table 1.
Bleeding symptoms in hemophilia carriers and normal women.

Clinical features	Carriers (%)	Controls (%)
Heavy menstrual bleeding	70	5
Cutaneous bruising	65	40
Oral cavity bleeding	50	25
Post-surgical bleeding	48	9
Hematomas	35	8
Postpartum bleeding	30	8
Hemarthrosis	18	0

Taken from the study of Paroskie [5].

Table 2.
Clinical traits related to hemorrhages in hemophilia carriers and normal women.

what would be expected, laboratory results do not always correlate with the clinical picture. A comparison of FVIII:C/FIX:C levels, hemoglobin, platelets, and fibrinogen between symptomatic hemophilia carriers and asymptomatic carriers did not reveal significant differences, yet a subgroup of carriers with factor levels within the lower normal range exhibited increased blood symptoms [14].

Srivaths et al. compared the bleeding complications in adolescents and adults and found that anemia and gynecologic procedures/surgeries were less frequent in adolescents likely because of an early detection [15]. On the other hand, in the case of HB due to Hemophilia B Leyden mutation (c.-22T>C) in the promotor of *F9* gene, there is a physiological mechanism that tends to normalize the FIX plasma levels according to age, which is mainly mediated by growth hormones rather than androgens that may ameliorate the bleeding symptoms in patients and female carriers [16].

2.4 Impact on women's health

The time between the start of bleeding symptoms and the diagnosis of a FVIII/FIX deficiency is often prolonged. Di Michele et al. reported that the mean period of diagnosis for hemophilia carriers with severe FVIII/FIX deficiency was 8.5 months compared to 2 months for similarly affected males; but if the deficiency was moderate, the diagnosis was delayed for 48 months compared to 4 months for similarly affected men [6].

The most common symptom, HMB, can have a significant impact on quality of life, missed days at work/school, iron deficiency anemia, need for hospitalization or blood transfusions, and higher costs in medical care [7]. Delayed diagnosis situates affected women at risk for co-morbidity and even mortality depending on the clinical context; this is why the carrier status and the percentage of clotting factor should be determined, and a proper genetic counseling should be offered [15].

2.5 Treatment

Dose, intervals, and duration for treatment depend on the clinical situation, effectiveness, and laboratory test results [7]. The treatment may include tranexamic acid, oral contraceptive pills (in some HMB), or factor VIII/IX [7, 15]. Hemostatic plans for hemophilia carriers with severe or mild FVIII/FIX deficiency should be noticed among primary care physicians and specialists in gynecology/obstetrics, hematology, orthopedics, clinical genetics, etc. Although each patient requires a personalized management, here we describe general guidelines for the treatment of the main hemorrhagic disorders in women:

2.5.1 HMB

Adolescents and women with HMB often respond well to standard therapies such as combined oral contraception pills, progestin-only pills, intrauterine devices, or antifibrinolytics such as aminocaproic acid or tranexamic acid. These therapies are warranted as the two key mechanisms in HMB are excessive local fibrinolytic mechanisms and inhibition of platelet function [7].

2.5.2 During pregnancy

The management of a hemophilia carrier should be coordinated among the hematologist, obstetrician, and anesthetist. During pregnancy, plasma levels of von Willebrand factor (VWF) and FVIII may rise sufficiently to permit safe hemostasis without exogenous hemostatic support, but they should be re-examined at 32–34 weeks of pregnancy; if the levels are less than 50% and more particularly less than 30% of the reference ranges, DDAVP or FVIII concentrates may be used. In pregnancy, FIX levels do not rise [17]. The use of DDAVP in symptomatic carriers of FVIII deficiency is controversial because the prescriber's information advises that the drug is contraindicated with lactation and recommends precaution during pregnancy. This drug has been used in the first and second trimester in 27 symptomatic carriers without adverse events [18]. Moreover, symptomatic carriers with factor levels less than 50% should receive a recombinant factor to prevent bleeding at delivery or spinal anesthesia [19]. Determination of fetal sex and prenatal hemophilia testing in any at-risk pregnancy are essential for planning the safe delivery of an affected female.

DDAVP is also indicated for HA patients with factor VIII coagulant activity levels greater than 5%. Intravenous dose is 0.3 μg/kg IV over 15–30 minutes (for pre-op, 30 minutes before the procedure). Intranasal administration is indicated for patients with FVIII levels >5% at a dose of 50 μg (if the patient's weight is <50 kg) or 300 μg (if weight ≥ 50 kg) 2 h before any surgical procedure [20].

2.6 Recommended integral management

Management of females represents a special challenge due to the risk of menorrhagia or postpartum bleeding, the large proportion (almost 40%) of unaware hemophilia carriers, and the medical inexperience of hemophilia in women.

The successful management in symptomatic hemophilia carriers requires the coordination of hematology, obstetrics/gynecology, orthopedics, and the coagulation laboratory as well as a complete education of the hemophilia carriers with the aim of providing them the best available information on the risk of bleeding, genetic implications in the offspring, reproductive options, and antenatal management of the affected offspring and mother [19].

3. von Willebrand disease in women

3.1 Generalities

VWD is the most common inherited bleeding disorder with a worldwide prevalence of 1% [21], associated with mucocutaneous and postoperative bleeding that is caused by a qualitative or quantitative defect of the VWF [22], a glycoprotein that participates in primary and secondary hemostasis via platelet adhesion at the site of the endothelial injury and platelet aggregation with the formation of the platelet plug, not to mention its role in transporting and stabilizing the FVIII [23].

VWD does not present sex, ethnic, or geographic predilection; however, the number of symptomatic women is greater than that of men in most populations (ratio 2:1) due to menstrual and delivery bleeding disorders [24]. The International Society on Thrombosis and Hemostasis (ISTH) recognizes six types of VWD [25] depending on the amount and functional activity of VWF. There can be a partial or total quantitative defect (type 1 and 3) or a qualitative defect (type 2) [26]. Moreover, type 2 VWD is subdivided into 4 variants (2A, 2B, 2M, and 2N) based on the details of the patient's phenotype [27].

3.2 Genetic aspects

The *VWF* gene, also known as *VWD*, is located at 12p13.3 and has a length of 178 kilobases (kb), and its 52 exons are transcribed into a 9 kb mRNA that encodes a pre-pro-VWF protein of 2813 amino acids whose different domains interact with other proteins and perform specific functions [28]. The expression of the *VWF* gene is limited to endothelial cells and megakaryocytes [29]. Different mutations cause quantitative (VWD types 1 and 3) or qualitative (type 2) defects in the VWF protein. VWD mostly has an autosomal dominant inheritance; only types 3 and 2N (in some cases type 2A) are inherited in an autosomal recessive manner [22].

3.3 Clinical features

Clinical manifestations of VWD could arise only when a hemostatic challenge occurs and include the following main symptoms:

- Excessive mucocutaneous bleeding.
- Hematoma with minimal trauma.
- Recurrent and prolonged epistaxis.
- Gingival hemorrhage.
- Prolonged bleeding after some dental procedure, surgery, or trauma.
- HMB (the most common symptom in women) or prolonged or excessive bleeding after delivery.

- Gastrointestinal bleeding, particularly in patients with type 2A VWD.
- Patients with type 3 and type 2N VWD may have hemarthroses due to a low level of FVIII [30].

3.4 Impact on women's health

HMB occurs in approximately 80% of cases and is associated with significant co-morbidity, namely iron deficiency anemia, stress, and reduction in the quality of life affecting daily activities; in addition, it entails higher costs in medical care [31]. There is evidence that women with VWD have higher rates of postpartum hemorrhage and transfusions at the time of delivery compared to healthy women [32].

Under normal conditions, postpartum hemorrhage is controlled due to the progressive increased activity of VWF and FVIII during pregnancy that reaches its maximum level at the time of delivery and subsequently decreases to a baseline level in approximately 1 month [32]. In VWD patients, the amount, functional activity, and behavior of VWF vary according to the disease's type and FVIII concentration **Figure 1** [33]. Although the function of the placenta may be impaired, there are inconsistent results about the risk of abortion in women with VWD [34].

Under normal conditions, a doubling of the levels of FVIII and VWF (VWF: Ag) and functional activity of the VWF (VWF: RCo) can be observed. Patients with severe VWD type 1 (increased clearance) do not show a significant increase in levels of VWF and FVIII. On the other hand, in type 1 there is a progressive increase in VWF levels; however, it is not as high as in normal conditions. In type 2A, the functional activity of VWF remains low due to the absence of high molecular weight multimers, and in type 2M the ratio of VWF: Ag/VWF: RCo is affected due to the low increase in VWF: RCo. In type 2N, FVIII remains reduced due to the inability of the VWF to bind to FVIII. Taken from Castaman [33].

3.5 Treatment

Because VWD is the most common cause of HMB, appropriate tests (measurement of VWF: Ag and VWF: RCo) should be performed to establish an accurate diagnosis and the specific treatment for the disease [35].

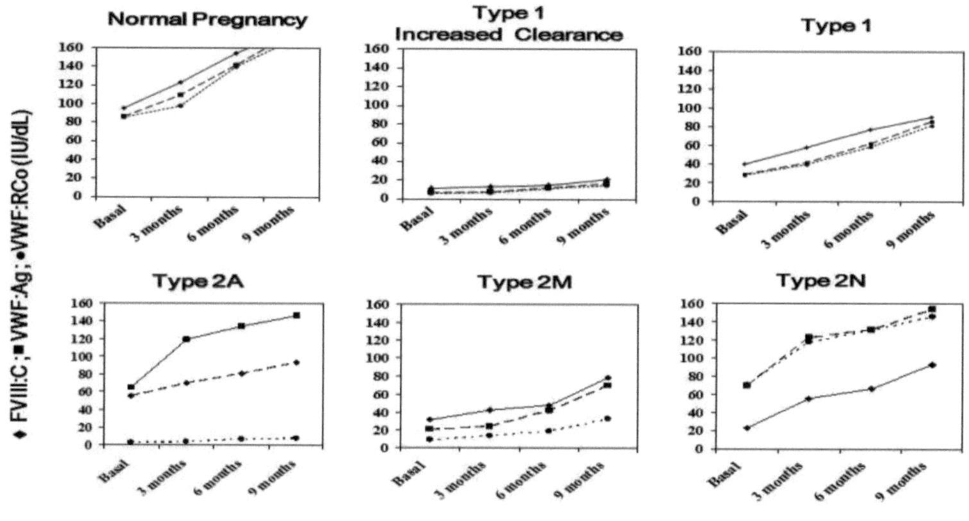

Figure 1.
Behavioral patterns of VWF and FVIII under normal conditions and in different VWD subtypes during pregnancy.

The treatment focuses on two central aspects: increasing the concentration of functional VWF available for hemostasis and providing complementary therapies to stabilize it [36]. DDAVP is administered intravenously or intranasally to increase plasmatic VWF through the release of endogenous VWF stored in Weibel-Palade bodies of endothelial cells. DDAVP is used in hemostatic challenges such as dental extractions and moderate nosebleeds or menorrhagia [36]. The administration of recombinant VWF is recommended in patients who do not respond to DDAVP or that require sustained levels of VWF in severe hemostatic challenges such as trauma and surgery [36]. Additional therapies include antifibrinolytic agents, amino-caproic acid, and tranexamic acid, which are recommended in mild to moderate bleedings. They are often used as adjunctive therapy in addition to concentrates of DDAVP or VWF in surgery or delivery [36].

3.6 Recommended integral management

Management in women presents a special challenge due to HMB and possible complications during pregnancy [37]. The successful management of pregnancy involves the coordination of obstetrics, anesthesia, and the coagulation laboratory that monitors levels of VWF: RCo and FVIII:C [37].

4. Platelet disorders

4.1 Idiopathic thrombocytopenic purpura (ITP)

4.1.1 Generalities

Idiopathic thrombocytopenic purpura or immune thrombocytopenia (ITP) is the most common acquired blood disorder. In this disease, autoantibodies against platelets render them susceptible to rapid clearance from the circulation [38–40]. Although the mechanism of origin of these antibodies is unknown, they belong to the gamma-globulin fraction expressed on platelet membranes and destroy the platelets [41–43] via their interaction with certain surface glycoproteins (GPs) identified as GP IIb-IIIa, GP Ib, and GP V [43]. The GP IIb-IIIa complex is the antigenic target in most patients. Platelets with antibodies are removed by splenic macrophages; however, their reactivation can lead to ineffective thrombopoiesis [40].

4.1.2 Genetic aspects

A positive family history is suggestive of hereditary thrombocytopenia. In addition to a presumptive autosomal dominant ITP, it has been found that the receptor for the Fc region of complexed immunoglobulin gamma (*FCGR2C*) predisposes to the disease [44, 45]. Several of their polymorphisms are related to the development of immunological reactions, but their contribution as a cause of ITP is still uncertain [46].

4.1.3 Clinical features

ITP can be acute or chronic and is characterized by (1) thrombocytopenia $<150 \times 10^9$ L^{-1} without other identifiable cause, (2) purpuric rash, and (3) normal function of bone marrow. Its approximate incidence is 3 to 8 per 100,000 children per year [43]. Acute ITP is frequent in children aged <10 years who have low platelet counts (usually 20,000 to 30×10^9 L^{-1}). The onset of signs and symptoms is often preceded by a viral illness. Chronic ITP affects mainly adolescents with platelet counts of 20-70×10^9 L^{-1}. Females are affected more frequently than males and are more likely to exhibit an underlying autoimmune disorder. Yet, the disease may be asymptomatic [43].

According to duration, ITP can be (1) newly diagnosed (<3 months), (2) persistent (between 3 and 6 months), or (3) chronic (>12 months). The clinical presentation can be (1) severe, patients with relevant bleeding, or requiring additional interventions or increased drug dose, or (2) refractory, severe clinical manifestations after splenectomy. Platelet counts define two types: (1) ≥100×10^9 L^{-1} measured on 2 occasions with more than 7 days between each sampling and (2) ≥30×10^9 L^{-1} and a greater than twofold increase in platelet count measured on 2 occasions >7 days apart [47].

Typical clinical presentation affects apparently healthy individuals; begins with easy bruising and purpuric rash [40]; and evolves to nasal, gingival, gastrointestinal tract, vaginal, urinary tract, retina, or conjunctivae bleedings. Bone marrow smears show normal or increased megakaryocytes, whereas plasma thrombopoietin levels are decreased. Patients with 10-20×10^9 L^{-1} of platelet counts are at increased risk for intracranial hemorrhage (ICH) [43].

4.1.4 Impact on women's health

About 7% of pregnancies or 1-10 in 10,000 pregnant women are diagnosed with gestational ITP (<150×10^9 L^{-1} of platelet count) generally in the first trimester [48, 49]. Only near 30% requires treatment and support from a multidisciplinary team [39, 50]. Recommended first-line therapy is intravenous immunoglobulin or corticosteroids, which have similar efficacy for platelet count increase. The latter may have mild toxicity for the mother and fetus, but usual adverse effects include weight gain, hyperglycemia, and hypertension [39].

4.1.5 Treatment

The pharmacologic management of acute ITP continues being controversial, because in approximately 80% of patients the disease is self-limited and disappears in the first 6 months after diagnosis without medication. For the 20% of patients who progress to the chronic type [43], prednisone at a standard dose of 1 mg/kg/day for 2–4 weeks is the first choice drug [39]. Yet, a randomized clinical trial has shown that it is better to use high-dose pulsed dexamethasone (40 mg/day for 4 days) than standard prednisone therapy in adult patients with immune thrombocytopenia [51].

4.1.6 Recommended integral management

Integral management of a patient with ITP is based on support measures (reduce physical activity, wear protective head-gear, adapt protective padding to the crib, avoid medications that affect platelets, and keep a constant evaluation and dental care) sometimes complemented with pharmacological and surgical treatment [43]. Patients require consulting a hematologist.

4.2 Bernard-Soulier syndrome

4.2.1 Generalities

Bernard-Soulier syndrome (BSS) results from a deficiency of platelet glycoprotein protein Ib (GPIb), which mediates the initial interaction of platelets with the subendothelial components via the von Willebrand protein. It is a rare but severe bleeding disorder in which platelets do not aggregate in response to ristocetin. Platelets from BSS patients lack a major surface membrane glycoprotein complex called GPIb-IX-V that functions as a receptor for VWF and whose absence causes giant platelets [52]. This complex is the initial contact for adhesion of platelets in damaged vessels, mediates the interaction with VWF (GPIb-IX-V/VWF), and interacts with the platelet cytoskeleton [52, 53]. The GPIb-IX-V complex comprises GPIbα, GPIbβ, GPIX, and GPV proteins whose assemblage forms the receptor [54].

4.2.2 Genetic aspects

BSS usually results from autosomal recessive mutations in *GP1BA*, *GP1BB*, and *GP9* genes that code for 3/4 proteins of the GPIb-IX-V complex (mutations in the 4th gene involved, *GP5*, are unreported) [52, 54]. Compound heterozygous patients outnumber homozygous patients. Only a few cases result from autosomal dominant mutations [55]. Although BSS carriers are usually asymptomatic with normal platelet counts, sometimes they show slightly enlarged platelets, slightly decreased GPIb-IX-V complex expression, and/or a moderately reduced ristocetin response [55, 56].

4.2.3 Clinical and hematological features

Clinical presentation of BSS is characterized by epistaxis, gingival and cutaneous bleeding, hemorrhages post trauma, prolonged skin bleeding time, thrombocytopenia, and large platelets. Patients often suffer from mucocutaneous bleedings of different severity [54]. In females, it can be associated with severe menorrhagia [52]. Typically, platelet counts are low, and the platelets are so large (often the size of red blood cells) that they may be missed on blood counts because most automatic counters do not count them as platelets [40]. The clinical laboratory assessment of GPIb-IX-V/VWF interaction with platelets reveals impaired platelet agglutination after stimulation with ristocetin [52, 54, 57].

4.2.4 Impact on women's health

Some women with BSS require oral contraceptive treatment for menorrhagia and even platelet transfusions in cases of severe bleeding [57]. Generally, pregnancies of patients with BSS are not complicated [58]. However, if during the delivery the patient presents severe bleeding, platelet transfusions or hysterectomy can be performed to control it [59].

4.2.5 Treatment

Usually, platelet transfusions are effective as BSS treatment; the inconvenience is the alloantibody development against GpIb [56]. Transfusions must be used only for severe bleeding and emergencies [40]. Also, the use of DDAVP, epsilon-aminocaproic acid (EACA), and recombinant factor VIIa (rVIIa) has been approved as an effective therapy for some patients [56].

4.2.6 Recommended integral management

BSS care is generally based on support measures only, inclusive for dental care. Actually, most patients do not require medication. The use of antiplatelet treatment must be avoided, and a hematologist should be consulted for its prescription [60].

4.3 Glanzmann thrombasthenia

4.3.1 Generalities

Glanzmann thrombasthenia (GT) is a rare dysfunction of the platelet integrin receptor CD41 (GPIIb/IIIa complex) that prevents the formation of aggregates in response to many agents, except for ristocetin [40, 56]. There are two GT types according to the functionality of the GP IIb/IIIa complex; type I is caused by the total absence of the GP IIb/IIIa complex and exhibits a more severe phenotype; type II is usually milder because some of the GP IIb/IIIa complexes are functional [40].

4.3.2 Genetic aspects

GT is an autosomal recessive disorder due to diverse mutations of the multi-subunit GpIIb/IIIa complex [56, 61–63]. The carriers or heterozygotes are asymptomatic, although they show a 50% reduction in the number of GpIIb/IIIa molecules [56]. *ITGA2B* and *ITGB3* genes code for proteins GPIIb and GPIIIa, respectively, and both are located at 17q21 [64]. GT is frequent in regions where consanguineous marriages are common [65, 66].

4.3.3 Clinical features

Clinical manifestations are variable in severity and frequency and depend on the genotype. Bleeding symptoms are present in patients homozygous or compound heterozygous for GPIIb/IIIa mutations [67]. As a minimum symptom, the patients have lifelong mucosal bleeding [56]. The bleeding (epistaxis, gingival hemorrhage, and menorrhagia) can be frequent, severe, and sometimes fatal [62, 68]. Severe epistaxis is common, mainly in childhood. Some patients only had bruising. Less commonly, gastrointestinal bleeding and hematuria have been observed [69]. The platelet count, morphology, and size are normal [56].

4.3.4 Impact on women's health

The transfusion history of red cell and/or platelet is frequent. Affected women are at risk of severe HMB and bleeding during pregnancy and delivery [69].

4.3.5 Treatment

The standard treatment for continuous bleeding has been platelet transfusions, especially for patients refractory to local measures and/or antifibrinolytic drugs [70]. However, the efficacy of platelet transfusion is limited by alloantibodies against platelets [56]. Several authors of clinical trials recommend the use of rFVIIa in the management of intractable epistaxis. It has been documented that this agent is effective in the management of bleeding or during surgeries at doses from 120 to 300 μg/kg [71, 72].

4.3.6 Recommended integral management

GT is a hemorrhagic lifelong disorder that requires integral support measures. Most patients have a history of transfusions indicated for severe bleeding [40, 67]. Fortunately, the prognosis of patients is good due to supportive care, and the disease has limited effect on their daily lives [69]. Dental and hematological advice is recommended.

5. Rare bleeding disorders (RBDs) in pregnancy and postpartum

5.1 Generalities

RBDs account for 3–5% of all inherited coagulation conditions and are characterized by a wide variability of bleeding symptoms that range from mild to severe in individuals affected by the same disorder. Most commonly, mucocutaneous bleeding and post-surgery hemorrhage are observed. Affected women usually suffer from menorrhagia, spontaneous abortion, and bleeding after delivery [73]. Although most RBDs are autosomal recessive traits, some cases of FXI deficiency and hypo- and dysfibrinogenemia are autosomal dominant. According to the epidemiological data of the World Federation of Hemophilia (WFH) and European Network of the Rare Bleeding Disorders (EN-RBDs), the prevalence of each deficiency among the total affected population is as follows: FVII (39%), FXI (26%), Fibrinogen, FV and FX (8–9%), FXIII (6%), combined FV + FVIII (3%), and FII (1%) [73].

Medical management and treatment of the RBSs are suboptimal because of their very low frequency. As a result, affected individuals received delayed diagnosis, incomplete laboratory testing, and limited treatment options. Standardization of coagulation assays, global clotting assays, and genomic sequencing promises to improve the diagnosis of RBDs, but there is still a long gap to overcome [1]. **Table 3** shows a general scope of the physiological characteristics, symptoms, and impact of the RBDs.

Deficiency	Plasma level (μg/mL)	Bleeding symptoms	Laboratory diagnosis	Prevalence	Gene (chromosome)
Fibrinogen	1500–4000	Umbilical cord, hemarthrosis, mucosal tract, menorrhagia, first trimester abortion, CNS Venous, and arterial thromboembolism are reported	*Afibrinogenemia:* APTT↑↑, PT↑↑, TT↑↑, *dys-hypofibrinogenemia*: APTT↑, PT↑↑, TT↑↑	1:1,000,000	*FGA, FGB,* and *FGG* (4q28)
F II	100	Umbilical cord, hemarthrosis, and mucosal tract	APTT↑↑, PT↑ TT normal	1:2,000,000	*F2* (11p11-q12)
F V	10	Mucosal tract and postoperative	APTT↑, PT↑, TT normal	1: 1,000,000	*F5* (1q24.2)
F VII	0.13–1.0	Mucosal tract, hemarthrosis, hematomas, and neonatal CNS hemorrage	APTT normal, PT↑, TT normal	1: 500,000	*F7* (13q34)
F X	10	Umbilical cord, hemarthrosis, hematomas, and CNS hemorrhages	APTT↑, PT↑, TT normal	1: 1,000,000	*F10* (13q34)
F XI	3–6	Oral cavity, post-traumatic, and postoperative	APTT↑, ↑T, PT normal, TT normal	1: 1,000,000	*F11* (4q35.2)

Deficiency	Plasma level (μg/mL)	Bleeding symptoms	Laboratory diagnosis	Prevalence	Gene (chromosome)
F XIII	10–20	Umbilical cord, spontaneous CNS hemorrhages, miscarriages, and abnormal scarring	APTT normal, PT normal, TT normal specific FXIII assay	1: 2,000,000	*F13A1* (6p24-p25) *F13B* (1q31-q32.1)
FV + FVIII	As for each factor	Mucosal tract and postoperative	APTT↑, PT↑, TT normal	1: 1,000,000	*LMAN1* (18q21.3-q22) *MCFD2* (2p21-p16.3)
VKCFD	As for each factor	Umbilical cord, CNS hemorrhages, and postoperative (children may show skeletal abnormalities)	APTT↑, PT↑↑, TT normal	<50 families	*GGCX* (2p12) *VKORC1* (16p11.2)

CNS, central nervous system; APTT, activated partial thromboplastin time; PT, prothrombin time. Taken from Castaman and Linari [73].

Table 3.
Clinical symptoms and laboratory/molecular diagnosis in rare bleeding disorders (RBDs).

5.2 RBDs in pregnancy, delivery, and puerperium

Women with RBDs require especial medical treatment and care. In addition to common bleeding symptoms, they may also experience gynecological bleeding and are at increased risk of hemorrhagic ovarian cysts, endometriosis, and endometrial hyperplasia polyps and fibroids. Pregnancy and childbirth in women with RBDs are real clinical challenges; miscarriages, bleeding during pregnancy, and postpartum hemorrhage are frequent and may represent severe clinical complications [74].

There has been a higher risk of diverse obstetric complications reported in women with RBDs; miscarriage and placental abruption resulting in fetal loss or preterm delivery are rather common in women deficient in fibrinogen or factor XIII (FXIII) [1].

To resolve the clinical complications of women with RBDs, it is important to consider the behavior of the clotting factors in normal conditions and their tendency to increase during pregnancy that has been attributed to the increase of estrogen concentrations, especially in the third trimester (fibrinogen, FVII, FVIII, FX, FXII, FXIII, and VWF). Other factors (FII, V, IX, and XIII) increase slightly or remain unchanged while FXI is the only factor that decreases during pregnancy [75].

6. Conclusion

Inherited bleeding disorders may seriously impact the women's quality of life through their detrimental effects on academic, professional, and social life. Long-lasting HMB causes iron deficiency anemia with consequences on physical and mental well-being. Medical care for women with bleeding disorders is lacking in many countries and there may be cultural taboos and obstacles preventing women from seeking help, specifically for menstrual problems, which may lead to marital disharmony and possibly fertility problems. Caregivers are often unaware about bleeding disorders in women, and therefore, even when women do seek help, the diagnosis is often neglected and appropriated treatment is not provided. In addition, bleeding disorders in women have negative consequences on the nutrition and well-being of their children. Early identification of young girls and women with HMB for managing their menstruation and iron deficiency is crucial in improving women's health in general [1].

Acknowledgements

We are grateful to Dr. Horacio Rivera for his valuable suggestions in the edition of the document. We dedicate this work to the Federación de Hemofilia de la República Mexicana, A.C., and we deeply appreciate their financial support for the publication.

Conflict of interest

All the authors declare that there is no conflict of interest regarding their contribution to this chapter.

Appendices and nomenclature

BSS	Bernard-Soulier syndrome
DDAVP	1-deamino-8-D-arginine vasopressin, denominated as desmopressin
EACA	epsilon-aminocaproic acid
FCGRC2	receptor for the Fc region of complexed immunoglobulin gamma
FIGO	The International Federation of Gynecology and Obstetrics
FIX:C	factor IX procoagulant activity
FVIII:C	factor VIII procoagulant activity
FXIII	factor XIII protein
F8	factor 8 gene
F9	factor 9 gene
GPIb	platelet glycoprotein protein Ib
GPs	platelet surface glycoproteins
GT	Glanzmann thrombasthenia
HA	hemophilia A
HB	hemophilia B
HMB	heavy menstrual bleeding
ICH	Intracranial hemorrhage
ISTH	International Society on Thrombosis and Hemostasis
ITP	idiopathic thrombocytopenic purpura or immune thrombocytopenia
IVIg	Intravenous immunoglobulin
Kb	Kilobases
PAI-1	plasminogen activator inhibitor
PBAC	pictorial blood assessment chart
PPH	postpartum hemorrhage
RBDs	rare bleeding disorders
rVIIa	recombinant factor VIIa

VWD	von Willebrand disease
VWF	von Willebrand factor
VWF:Ag	antigen test of the VWF used to measure the amount of VWF
VWF:RCo	a ristocetin cofactor test used to measure functional activity of the VWF

Author details

Ana-Rebeca Jaloma-Cruz[1*], Isaura-Araceli González-Ramos[2], Diana Ornelas-Ricardo[3], Clara-Ibet Juárez-Vázquez[2] and Hilda Luna-Záizar[4]

1 Genetics Division, Biomedical Research Center of Occident, Mexican Institute of Social Security, Guadalajara, Jalisco, Mexico

2 Genetics Department, Institute of Biological Sciences, Medicine Faculty, Autonomous University of Guadalajara, Guadalajara, Jalisco, Mexico

3 PhD Program on Human Genetics, University Center of Health Sciences, University of Guadalajara, Guadalajara, Jalisco, Mexico

4 Department of Chemistry, University Center of Exact Sciences and Engineering, University of Guadalajara, Guadalajara, Jalisco, Mexico

*Address all correspondence to: arjaloma@gmail.com

IntechOpen

© 2018 The Author(s). Licensee IntechOpen. This chapter is distributed under the terms of the Creative Commons Attribution License (http://creativecommons.org/licenses/by/3.0), which permits unrestricted use, distribution, and reproduction in any medium, provided the original work is properly cited.

References

[1] Kadir RA, James AH. Reproductive Health in Women with Bleeding Disorders. World Federation of Hemophilia, Treatment of Hemophilia Series; 2009. Vol. 48. pp. 1-13. Available from: http://www.wfh.org

[2] Hermans C, Kulkarni R. Women with bleeding disorders. Hemophilia. 2018;**24**:29-36. DOI: 10.1111/hae.13502

[3] Fraser IS, Critchley HOD, Broder M. The FIGO recommendations on terminologies and definitions for normal and abnormal uterine bleeding. Seminars in Reproductive Medicine. 2011;**29**:383-390. DOI: 10.1055/s-0031-1287662

[4] Higham JM, O'Brien PM, Shaw RW. Assessment of menstrual blood loss using a pictorial chart. British Journal of Obstetrics and Gynaecology. 1990;**97**:734-739. DOI: 10.1111/j.1471-0528.1990.tb16249.x

[5] Paroskie A, Gailani D, DeBraun MR. A cross-sectional study of bleeding phenotype in haemophilia A carriers. British Journal of Haematology. 2015;**170**:223-228. DOI: 10.1111/bjh.13423

[6] Di Michele DM, Gibb C, Lefkowitz JM. Severe and moderate haemophilia A and B in US females. Haemophilia. 2014;**20**:e136-e143. DOI: 10.1111/hae.12364

[7] Staber J, Croteau SE, Davis J. The spectrum of bleeding in women and girls with haemophilia B. Haemophilia. 2018;**24**:180-185. DOI: 10.1111/hae.13376

[8] Pavlova A, Brondke H, Müsebeck J. Molecular mechanisms underlying hemophilia A phenotype in seven females. Journal of Thrombosis and Haemostasis. 2009;**7**:976-982. DOI: 10.1111/j.1538-7836.2009.03346.x

[9] Khan MTS, Naz A, Ahmed J. Diagnosis and phenotypic assessment of Pakistani haemophilia B carriers. Pakistan Journal of Medical Sciences. 2017;**33**:738-742. DOI: 10.12669/pjms.333.12496

[10] Olsson A, Ljung R, Hellgren M. Phenotype and genotype comparisons in carriers of haemophilia A. Haemophilia. 2016;**22**:e235-e237. DOI: 10.1111/hae.12928

[11] Bernard W, Lambert C, Henrard S. Screening of haemophilia carriers in moderate and severe haemophilia A and B: Prevalence and determinants. Haemophilia. 2018;**24**:e142-e144. DOI: 10.1111/hae.13468

[12] Lavaut K. Importancia del diagnóstico de portadoras en familias con antecedentes de hemofilia. Revista Cubana de Hematologia e Inmunología y Hemoterapia. 2014;**30**:108-113. ISBN 0864-0289

[13] Olsson A, Hellgren M, Berntorp E. Association between bleeding tendency and health-related quality of life in carriers of moderate and severe haemophilia. Haemophilia. 2015;**21**:742-746. DOI: 10.1111/hae.12796

[14] Olsson A, Hellgren M, Berntorp E. Clotting factor level is not a good predictor of bleeding in carriers of haemophilia A and B. Blood Coagulation & Fibrinolysis. 2014;**25**:471-475. DOI: 10.1097/MBC.0000000000000083

[15] Srivaths LV, Zhang QC, Byams VR. Differences in bleeding phenotype and provider interventions in postmenarchal adolescents when compared to adult women with bleeding disorders and heavy menstrual bleeding. Haemophilia. 2018;**24**:63-69. DOI: 10.1111/hae.13330

[16] Hildyard C, Keeling D. Effect of age on factor IX levels in symptomatic carriers of haemophila B Leyden. British Journal of Haematology. 2015;**169**: 448-449. DOI: 10.1111/bjh.13223

[17] Street AM, Ljung R, Lavery SA. Management of carriers and babies with haemophilia. Haemophilia. 2008;**14**:181-187. DOI: 10.1111/j.1365-2516.2008.01721.x

[18] Mannucci PM. Use of desmopressin (DDAVP) during early pregnancy in factor VIII-deficient women. Blood. 2005;**105**:3382. DOI: 10.1182/blood-2004-11-4472

[19] Lavee O, Kidson-Gerber G. Update on inherited disorders of haemostasis and pregnancy. Obstetric Medicine. 2016;**9**:64-72. DOI: 10.1177/1753495X15624307

[20] Medscape Drug Reference [Internet]; Lundberg. 2018. Available from: https://reference.medscape.com/drug/ddavp-stimate-noctiva-desmopressin-342819 [Accessed: July 7, 2018]

[21] Pikta M, Zemtsovskaja G, Bautista H. Preclinical evaluation of a semi-automated and rapid commercial electrophoresis assay for von Willebrand factor multimers. Journal of Clinical Laboratory Analysis. 2018;**32**:e22416. DOI: 10.1002/jcla.22416

[22] De Jong A, Eikenboom J. Developments in the diagnostic procedures for von Willebrand disease. Journal of Thrombosis and Haemostasis. 2016;**14**:449-460. DOI: 10.1111/jth.13243

[23] Stockschlaeder M, Schneppenheim R, Budde U. Update on von Willebrand factor multimers: Focus on high-molecular-weight multimers and their role in hemostasis. Blood Coagulation & Fibrinolysis. 2014;**25**:206-216. DOI: 10.1097/MBC.00000000000 00065

[24] Lillicrap D. von Willebrand disease: Advances in pathogenetic understanding diagnosis and therapy. Blood. 2013;**122**:3735-3740. DOI: 10.1182/asheducation-2013.1.254

[25] Favaloro EJ, Bonar RA, Meiring M. Evaluating errors in the laboratory identification of von Willebrand disease in the real world. Thrombosis Research. 2014;**134**:393-403. DOI: 10.1016/j.thromres.2014.05.020

[26] Lehner S, Ekhlasi-Hundrieser M, Detering C. A 12.3-kb duplication within the VWF gene in pigs affected by von Willebrand disease type 3. G3 (Bethesda). 2018;**8**:577-585. DOI: 10.1534/g3.117.300432

[27] Nichols WL, Hultin MB, James AH. von Willebrand disease (VWD): Evidence based diagnosis management guidelines, the National Heart, Lung and Blood Institute (NHLBI), expert Panel report (USA). Haemophilia. 2008;**14**:171-232. DOI: 10.1111/j.1365-2516.2007.01643.x

[28] VWF von Willebrand factor [*Homo sapiens* (human)]—Gene—NCBI [Internet]. 2018. Available from: https://www.ncbi.nlm.nih.gov/gene/7450 [Accessed: July 10, 2018]

[29] Xiang Y, Hwa J. Regulation of VWF expression, and secretion in health and disease. Current Opinion in Hematology. 2016;**23**:288-293. DOI: 10.1097/MOH.0000000000000230

[30] Sharma R, Flood VH. Advances in the diagnosis and treatment of von Willebrand disease. Hematology. American Society of Hematology. Education Program. 2017;**1**:379-384. DOI: 10.1182/asheducation-2017.1.379

[31] Ragni MV, Machin N, Malec LM. von Willebrand factor for menorrhagia: A survey and literature review. Haemophilia. 2016;**22**:397-402. DOI: 10.1111/hae.12898

[32] James AH, Konkle BA, Kouides P. Postpartum von Willebrand factor levels in women with and without von Willebrand disease and implications for prophylaxis. Haemophilia. 2015;**21**: 81-87. DOI: 10.1111/hae.12568

[33] Castaman G. Changes of von Willebrand Factor during Pregnancy in Women with and without von Willebrand Disease. Mediterranean Journal of Hematology and Infectious Diseases. 2013;**5**:2013052. DOI: 10.4084/MJHID.2013.052

[34] Skeith L, Rydz N, O'Beirne M. Pregnancy loss in women with von Willebrand disease: A single-center pilot study. Blood Coagulation & Fibrinolysis. 2017;**28**:393-397. DOI: 10.1097/MBC.0000000000000620

[35] Lee C, Kadir A, Kouides P. Women with von Willebrand disease. In: Federici A, Lee C, editors. von Willebrand Disease: Basic and Clinical Aspects. 1st ed. Chichester: Wiley; 2011. pp. 174-185

[36] Ng CJ, Paola D, von Willebrand Disease J. Diagnostic strategies and treatment options. Pediatric Clinics of North America. 2018;**65**:527-541. DOI: 10.1016/j.pcl.2018.02.004

[37] Neff AT, Sidonio RF Jr. Management of VWD. Hematology. American Society of Hematology. Education Program. 2014;**2014**:536-541. DOI: 10.1182/asheducation 2014.1.536

[38] Ahn YS, Horstman LL. Idiopathic thrombocytopenic purpura: Pathophysiology and management. International Journal of Hematology. 2002;**76**:123-131. PMID: 12430912

[39] Lambert MP, Gernsheimer TB. Clinical updates in adult immune thrombocytopenia. Blood. 2017;**129**:2829-2835. DOI: 10.1182/blood-2017-03-754119

[40] Medscape Drug Reference. Platelet Disorders Overview of Platelet Disorders [Internet]. 2017. Available from: https://emedicine.medscape.com/article/201722-overview#showall [Accessed: July 24, 2018]

[41] Harrington WJ, Minnich V, Hollingsworth JW. Demonstration of a thrombocytopenic factor in the blood of patients with thrombocytopenic purpura. Journal of Laboratory and Clinical Medicine. 1951;**115**:636-645. PMID: 2187937

[42] Arimura G, Harrington WJ, Minnich V. The autoimmune thrombocytopenias. Progress in Hematology. 1956;**1**:166-192. PMID:13359508

[43] Chu YW, Korb J, Sakamoto KM. Idiopathic thrombocytopenic purpura. Pediatrics in Review. 2000;**21**:95-104. PMID: 10702324

[44] Breunis WB, van Mirre E, Bruin M. Copy number variation of the activating *FCGR2C* gene predisposes to idiopathic thrombocytopenic purpura. Blood. 2008;**111**:1029-1038. DOI: 10.1182/blood-2007-03-079913

[45] Online Mendelian Inheritance in Man (OMIM). Thrombocytopenic purpura autoimmune (OMIM 188030) [Internet]. 2009. Available from: https://www.omim.org/entry/188030#9 [Accessed: July 24, 2018]

[46] U.S. National Library of Medicine. Genetics Home Reference. Immune thrombocytopenia [Internet]. 2018. Available from: https://ghr.nlm.nih.gov/condition/immune-thrombocytopenia#genes [Accessed: July 25, 2018]

[47] Rodeghiero F, Stasi R, Gernsheimer T. Standardization of terminology, definitions and outcome criteria in immune thrombocytopenic purpura of adults and children: Report from an international working group. Blood. 2009;**113**:2386-2393. DOI: 10.1182/blood-2008-07-162503

[48] Kelton JG. Idiopathic thrombocytopenic purpura complicating pregnancy. Blood Reviews. 2002;**16**:43-46. DOI: 10.1054/blre.2001.0181

[49] American College of Obstetricians and Gynecologists. ACOG practice bulletin: Thrombocytopenia in pregnancy. Number 6, September 1999. Clinical management guidelines for obstetrician-gynecologists. International Journal of Gynecology & Obstetrics. 1999;**67**:117-128. PMID: 10636060

[50] Webert KE, Mittal R, Sigouin C. A retrospective 11-year analysis of obstetric patients with idiopathic thrombocytopenic purpura. Blood. 2003;**102**:4306-4311. DOI: 10.1182/blood-2002-10-3317

[51] Matschke J, Müller-Beissenhirtz H, Novotny J. A randomized trial of daily prednisone versus pulsed dexamethasone in treatment-naïve adult patients with immune thrombocytopenia: EIS 2002 Study. Acta Haematologica. 2016;**136**:101-107. DOI: 10.1159/000445420

[52] Lopez JA, Andrews RK, Afshar-Kharghan V. Bernard-Soulier syndrome. Blood. 1998;**91**:4397-4418. PMID: 9616133

[53] Andrews R, Berndt M, Lopez J. The glycoprotein Ib-IX-V complex. In: Michelson AD, editor. Platelets. 2nd ed. San Diego, CA: Academic Press; 2006. pp. 145-164

[54] Li R, Emsley J. The organizing principle of the platelet glycoprotein Ib-IX-V complex. Journal of Thrombosis and Haemostasis. 2013;**11**:605-614. DOI: 10.1111/jth.12144

[55] Noris P, Perrotta S, Bottega R. Clinical and laboratory features of 103 patients from 42 Italian families with inherited thrombocytopenia derived from the monoallelic Ala156Val mutation of GPIb alpha (Bolzano mutation). Haematologica. 2012;**97**:82-88. DOI: 10.3324/haematol.2011.050682

[56] Handin RI. Inherited platelet disorders. Hematology American Society of Hematology Education Program. 2005;**1**:396-402. DOI: 10.1182/asheducation-2005.1.396

[57] Savoia A, Pastore A, De Rocco D. Clinical and genetic aspects Bernard-Soulier syndrome: Searching for genotype/phenotype correlations. Haematologica. 2011;**96**:417-423. DOI: 10.3324/haematol.2010.032631

[58] Peng TC, Kickler TS, Bell WR. Obstetric complications in a patient with Bernard-Soulier syndrome. American Journal of Obstetrics and Gynecology. 1991;**165**:425-426. PMID: 1714677

[59] Peaceman AM, Katz AR, Laville M. Bernard-Soulier syndrome complicating pregnancy: A case report. Obstetrics and Gynecology. 1989;**73**:457-459. PMID: 2915873

[60] Medscape Drug Reference. Bernard-Soulier Syndrome Treatment & Management [Internet]. 2016. Available from: https://emedicine.medscape.com/article/954877-treatment [Accessed: July 24, 2018]

[61] D'Andrea G, Colaizzo D, Vecchione G. Glanzmann's thrombasthenia: Identification of 19 new mutations in 30 patients. Thrombosis and Haemostasis. 2002;**87**:1034-1042. PMID: 12083483

[62] Bellucci S, Caen J. Molecular basis of Glanzmann's thrombasthenia and current strategies in treatment. Blood Reviews. 2002;**16**:193-202. PMID: 12163005

[63] Nair S, Ghosh K, Kulkarni B. Glanzmann's thrombasthenia: Updated.

Platelets. 2002;**13**:387-393. DOI: 10.1080/0953710021000024394

[64] Rosenberg N, Yatuv R, Sobolev V. Major mutations in calf-1 and calf-2 domains of glycoprotein IIb in patients with Glanzmann thrombasthenia enable GPIIb/IIIa complex formation, but impair its transport from the endoplasmic reticulum to the Golgi apparatus. Blood. 2003;**101**:4808-4815. DOI: 10.1182/blood-2002-08-2452

[65] Newman PJ, Seligsohn U, Lyman S. The molecular genetic basis of Glanzmann thrombasthenia in the Iraqi-Jewish and Arab populations in Israel. Proceedings of the National Academy of Sciences of the United States of America. 1991;**88**:3160-3164. PMID: 2014236

[66] Toogeh G, Sharifian R, Lak M. Presentation and pattern of symptoms in 382 patients with Glanzmann thrombasthenia in Iran. American Journal of Hematology. 2004;**77**: 198-199. DOI: 10.1002/ajh.20159

[67] Franchini M, Favaloro EJ, Lippi G. Glanzmann thrombasthenia: An update. Clinica Chimica Acta. 2010;**411**:1-6. DOI: 10.1016/j.cca.2009.10.016

[68] Nurden AT, George JN. Inherited abnormalities of the platelet membrane: Glanzmann thrombasthenia, Bernard-Soulier syndrome, and other disorders. In: Hemostasis and Thrombosis, Basic Principles and Clinical Practice. 6th ed. Philadelphia: Lippincott, Williams & Wilkins; 2005. pp. 987-1010

[69] Nurden AT. Glanzmann thrombasthenia. Orphanet Journal of Rare Diseases. 2006;**6, 1**:10. DOI: 10.1186/1750-1172-1-10

[70] Poon MC, Zotz R, Di Minno G. Glanzmann's thrombasthenia treatment: A prospective observational registry on the use of recombinant human activated factor VII and other hemostatic agents. Seminars in Hematology. 2006;**43**:S33-S536. DOI: 10.1053/j.seminhematol.2005.11.009

[71] Valentino LA. Use of rFVIIa in 4 children with Glanzmann thromboasthenia. Journal of Pediatric Hematology/Oncology. 2006;**28**:653-658. DOI: 10.1097/01.mph.0000212993.49188.73

[72] Franchini M. The use of recombinant activated factor VII in platelet disorders: A critical review of the literature. Blood Transfusion. 2009;**7**:24-28. DOI: 10.2450/2008.0015-08

[73] Castaman G, Linari S. Diagnosis and treatment of von Willebrand disease and rare bleeding disorders. Journal of Clinical Medicine. 2017;**6**:1-18. DOI: 10.3390/jcm6040045

[74] Palla R, Peyvandy F, Shapiro AD. Rare bleeding disorders: Diagnosis and treatment. Review Series. Blood. 2015;**125**:2052-2061. DOI: 10.1182/blood-2014-08-532820

[75] Hellgren M. Hemostasis during normal pregnancy and puerperium. Seminars in Thrombosis and Hemostasis. 2003;**29**:125-130. DOI: 10.1159/000217305